THE EASY
MEDITERRANEAN DIET
MEAL PLAN

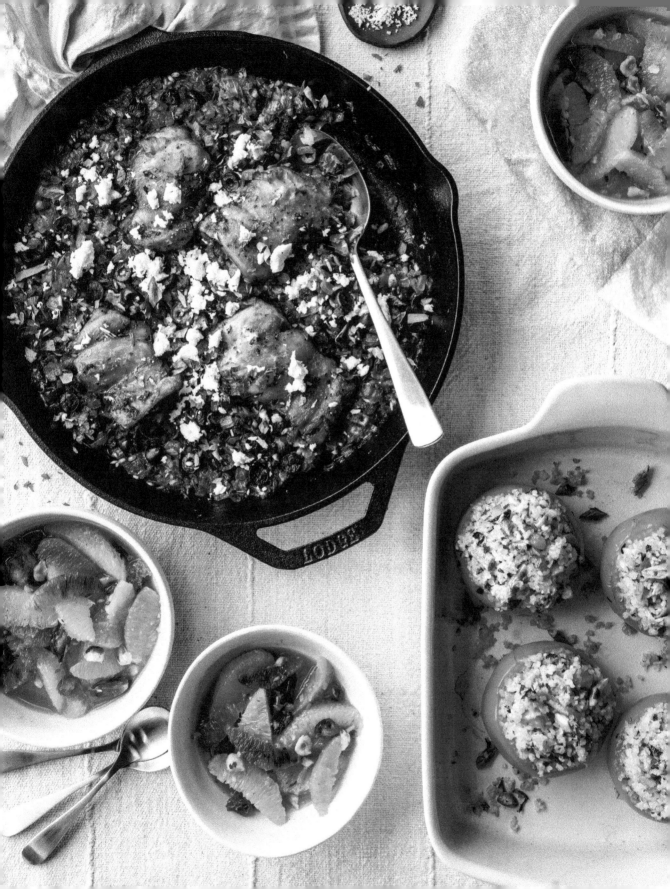

THE EASY MEDITERRANEAN DIET MEAL PLAN

4 WEEKS
to Jump-start Your Journey
to Lifelong Health

SUSAN ZOGHEIB, MHS, RD

ROCKRIDGE
PRESS

Interior and Cover Designer: Peatra Jariya
Art Producer: Karen Beard
Editor: Ada Fung
Production Manager: Oriana Siska
Production Editor: Melissa Edeburn

Cover photography © 2019 Thomas J. Story, Food Styling Karen Shinto, salmon © Nadine Greeff.

Interior photography © 2019 Thomas J. Story, Food Styling Karen Shinto, except pp. vi, viii, x, 18, 120, and 196 © Nadine Greeff

ISBN: Print 978-1-64152-630-2 | eBook 978-1-64152-631-9

To my boys—
Brian, Brycen, and Mason

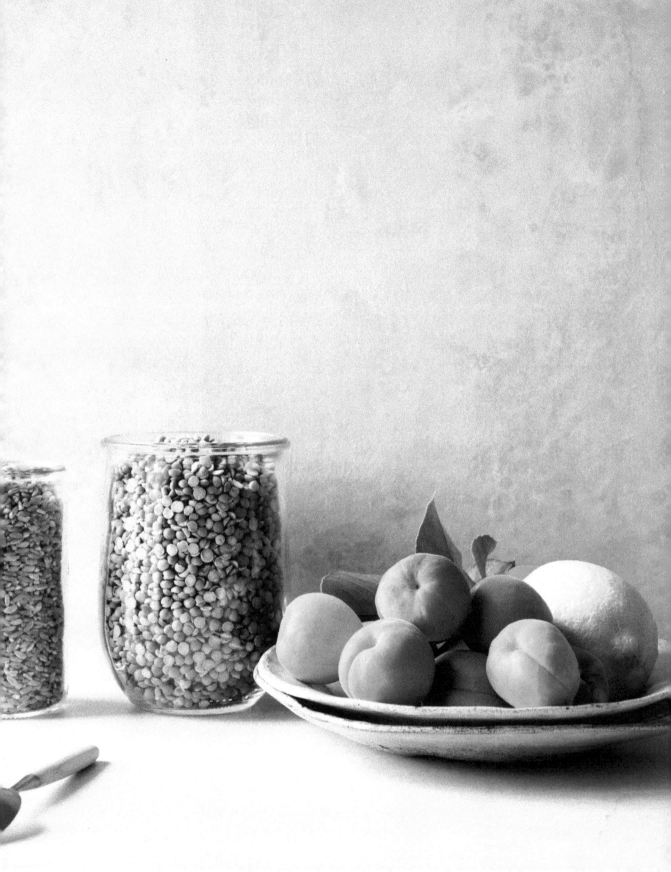

CONTENTS

Introduction   IX

PART ONE: THE MEDITERRANEAN DIET 101   1

CHAPTER 1: Mediterranean Diet Basics   3
CHAPTER 2: The Mediterranean Kitchen and Pantry   13

PART TWO: WEEKLY MEAL PLAN WITH RECIPES   19

CHAPTER 3: Week One Meal Plan and Recipes   21
CHAPTER 4: Week Two Meal Plan and Recipes   45
CHAPTER 5: Week Three Meal Plan and Recipes   67
CHAPTER 6: Week Four Meal Plan and Recipes   91
CHAPTER 7: After the Four-Week Plan   115

PART THREE: MEDITERRANEAN RECIPES FOR LIFE   121

CHAPTER 8: Breakfast and Brunch   123
CHAPTER 9: Fish and Shellfish   135
CHAPTER 10: Poultry and Lean Meat   147
CHAPTER 11: Vegetables, Grains, and Legumes   163
CHAPTER 12: Snacks and Sweets   179
CHAPTER 13: Dressings and Dips   187

Blank Meal Plan   197
Measurement Conversions   198
The Dirty Dozen and the Clean Fifteen™   199
References   200
Recipe Index   201
Index   203

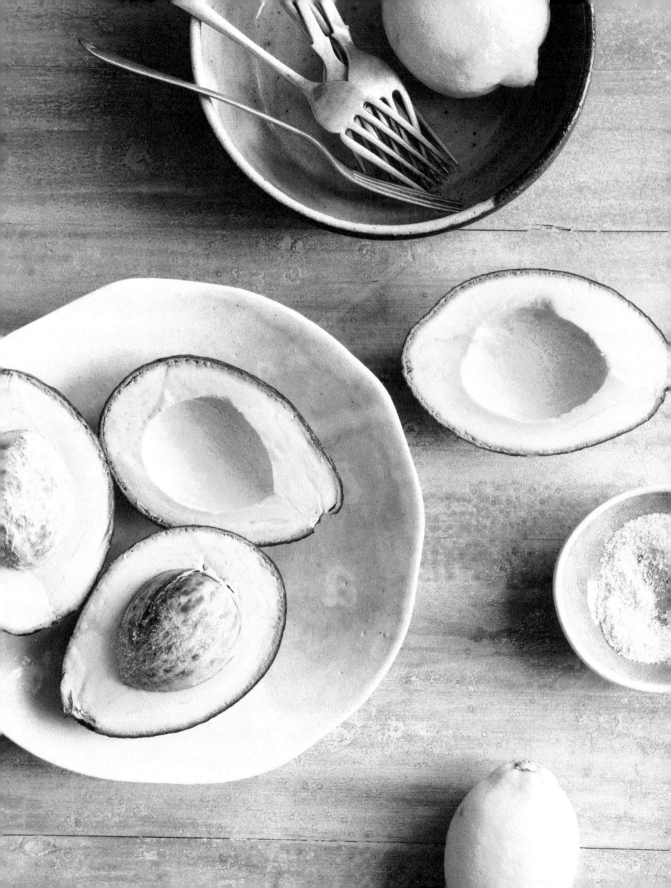

ꟼNTRODUCTION

I was born in the Middle East and grew up cooking and eating Mediterranean food. Much of my Lebanese upbringing revolved around the family dinner table. Far more than just a flat surface for dining, the kitchen table, for me, was and continues to be the heartbeat of my family. It's a place to gather, to talk, and to reconnect. Cozy and comfortable, our time at the kitchen table helped us come together and sit closer to one another. I loved these moments we shared as a family.

Tabbouleh, hummus, falafel, and shawarma, just to name a few, were some of my favorite staples growing up. To be from the land where these items were created is a true treat. Moreover, the Mediterranean climate made it easy for my family to grow fresh fruits and vegetables in our backyard.

The Mediterranean diet is not just a diet—it is a way of life. Although tasty plant proteins, delicious fish, occasional red meat, and plenty of fresh fruits and vegetables are hallmarks of the diet, you can also have your share of grains and even a glass of red wine, all while reaping major health benefits. The Mediterranean diet has been proven effective for weight loss, and it may even protect against disease and increase your life expectancy. I look forward to guiding you through the Mediterranean diet and starting this exciting journey with you for an overall healthy makeover.

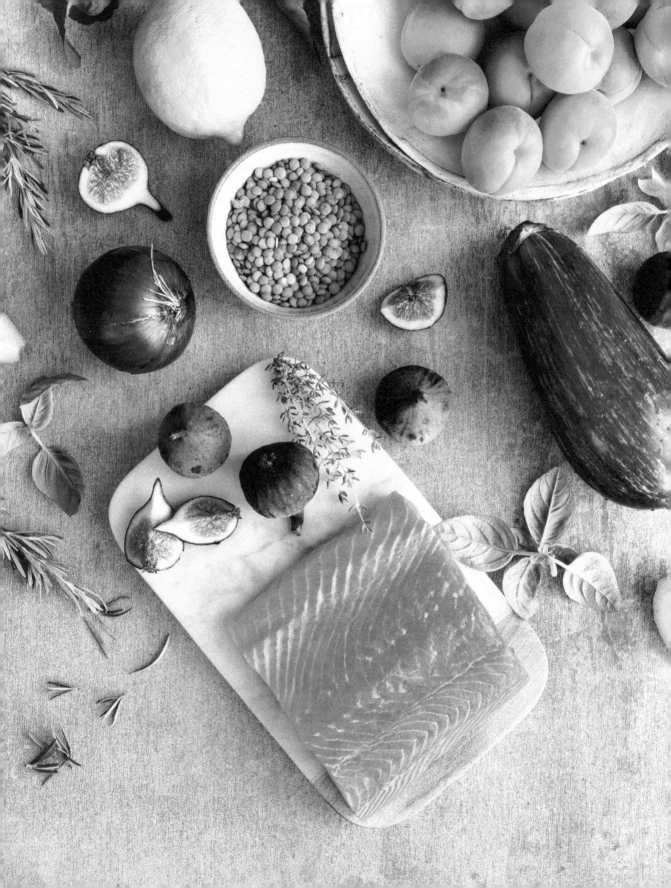

PART ONE

THE MEDITERRANEAN DIET 101

Starting a new diet and making a lifestyle change can be daunting, but rest assured—you are not alone on this journey. I believe that the best way to accomplish and sustain any lifestyle change is to prepare yourself by understanding it and what it takes to stick with it. From breaking down the nuts and bolts of Mediterranean eating and living to helping you set up your kitchen and pantry, this section will give you all the tools and resources you need to understand the Mediterranean diet. I will help you prepare to begin this diet and show you how to successfully maintain it for lifelong health.

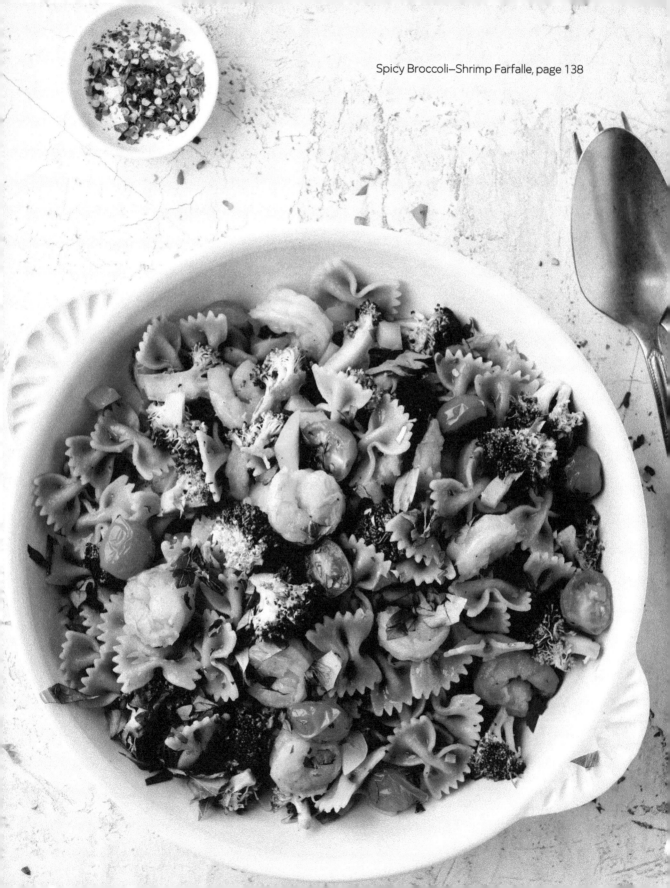

Spicy Broccoli–Shrimp Farfalle, page 138

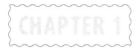
CHAPTER 1

Mediterranean Diet Basics

The Mediterranean diet has quickly become one of the world's most popular and most effective diets, but it is more than an eating plan: The Mediterranean diet is a lifestyle. In this chapter, I will provide you with an overview of the Mediterranean diet and give you the information and tips you need to kick off your healthy journey and stay on it. From experimenting with new spices and ingredients to making time to enjoy a meal with your family, you will soon feel confident in your new Mediterranean lifestyle.

WHAT IS THE MEDITERRANEAN DIET?

The Mediterranean diet is a generic concept based on the typical eating habits in the countries that border the Mediterranean Sea. From Turkey to Egypt to Portugal to France to Spain to Israel and beyond, the Mediterranean diet embodies the traditional ingredients and recipes used by 16 countries.

Dr. Ancel Keys, a Minnesota physiologist, first championed the health benefits of the Mediterranean diet in the 1960s. As the lead researcher on the Seven Countries Study, he determined that saturated fat was a major cause of heart disease but showed that even with up to 35 percent of its calories coming from fat, the Mediterranean diet, through its use of healthier fats, can protect against heart disease and benefit the body.

There is no one true "Mediterranean" diet, due to the diversity of religions, cultures, ethnicities, and agricultural practices across the region. However, some commonalities include the following:

- fruits, vegetables, whole grains, and olive oil eaten daily
- beans, legumes, and nuts eaten at least twice a week
- fish eaten at least twice a week
- moderate portions of sheep's milk cheese and yogurt eaten daily to weekly
- moderate portions of poultry and eggs eaten every two days or weekly
- limited red meat consumption
- drinking plenty of water
- wine in moderation—for women, no more than one (5-ounce) serving daily and for men, two (5-ounce) servings per day

SEVEN REASONS TO CHOOSE THE MEDITERRANEAN DIET

What's the hype with the Mediterranean diet? There are many reasons why this diet was ranked number one by the *US News & World Report* and is recommended for improved physical and mental health. With anti-inflammatory properties, realistic food goals, and inherent variety, this diet is considered one of the best to manage weight, lower the risk of cardiovascular disease, manage chronic illnesses related to obesity, and decrease stress. Here are some of the reasons to choose the Mediterranean diet:

Decrease the risk of heart disease. According to the AHA, the Mediterranean diet is the number one diet for the prevention of heart-related diseases. It can help decrease blood pressure, decrease the risk of heart attack and stroke, and reduce arterial inflammation, which is important because blocked arteries, or atherosclerosis, are the leading cause of death in the United States. The diet encourages the consumption of many fruits and vegetables, while limiting the consumption of red meat. The diet also focuses on fresh and natural ingredients, which have more vitamins and minerals than processed foods. These factors result in a diet high in heart-healthy nutrients and low in saturated fats and added sugars.

Control blood glucose levels. The Mediterranean diet has been shown to reduce the risk of diabetes and even prevent type 2 diabetes. The fiber in fruits, vegetables, whole grains, and legumes works to slow digestion, which in turn helps control spikes in your blood sugar levels. By balancing our

The Mediterranean Diet Pyramid

Scientific research has shown that adopting the Mediterranean diet plan, outlined in the pyramid chart below, provides a host of health benefits, including a lower risk for cancer and improved heart health.

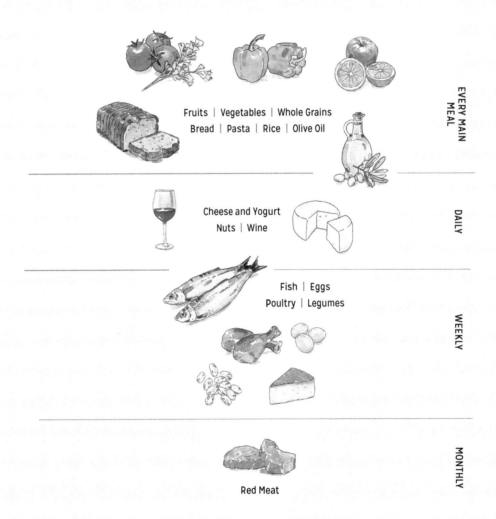

Fruits | Vegetables | Whole Grains
Bread | Pasta | Rice | Olive Oil

EVERY MAIN MEAL

Cheese and Yogurt
Nuts | Wine

DAILY

Fish | Eggs
Poultry | Legumes

WEEKLY

Red Meat

MONTHLY

consumption of simple carbs, such as sugars found naturally in fruits and dairy, with complex carbs like whole grains, protein, and healthy fats, digestion can be slowed down enough to properly utilize those carbohydrates and reduce insulin resistance.

Improve digestion. Fiber is an essential part of the diet, along with anti-inflammatory properties and nutrients that function as pre- and probiotics, which can create a more diverse gut microbiota and improve bowel function.

Manage and maintain body weight. The Mediterranean diet encourages quality meal times instead of a quick bite to eat; taking a walk to the nearest grocery store instead of driving; and reducing portions and eating slowly instead of overeating in haste. These factors, combined with the improved nutrient variety and decreased consumption of saturated fat, can help you reach a healthy body weight and maintain a diet that is sustainable.

Reduce inflammation. Omega-3 fatty acids have been shown to decrease inflammation, a primary culprit in several diseases including cardiovascular diseases, digestive disorders, joint pain, and more. The Mediterranean diet is full of foods rich in omega-3 fatty acids, like tuna, salmon, walnuts, and chia seeds. Research has found that eating these types of foods can help improve cholesterol levels, control weight, and decrease the risk of developing diabetes, Alzheimer's disease, and multiple types of cancer.

Improve brain function. The Mediterranean diet can improve the health of your brain and decrease the risks of Alzheimer's disease. Research has shown that healthy fats may contribute to the prevention of cognitive decline, and that there is a direct correlation between the consumption of fish and decreased prevalence of Alzheimer's.

Improve mood and decrease stress. Studies show that adherence to the Mediterranean diet can reduce the risk of depression and improve mood. This is likely because the diet encourages a lifestyle that pulls us away from hectic Westernized activities and focuses on family, exercise, and decreased time on media devices. It encourages family meal times, daily physical activity that is incorporated into daily tasks, and an active lifestyle. These factors can improve mood and overall mental health.

THE NUTS AND OLIVES OF THE MEDITERRANEAN DIET

The Mediterranean diet is not about restriction, and there is no one-diet-fits-all approach. However, here are a few general guidelines to follow when implementing the Mediterranean diet.

Increase fruit and vegetable intake. About half of your plate at each meal should consist of fruits or vegetables. For example, when eating a dish with a grain and meat or fish, make sure to include a side salad and maybe a piece of fruit. Or, when making a snack, have a fruit combined with a protein such as nut butter. These heart-healthy options are high in fiber and low in fat, making them ideal for heart health. They also include antioxidants like vitamins A, C, E, and K, which can reduce inflammation and the risk of clogged arteries.

Use whole grains regularly. Choosing whole-grain breads, pastas, or brown rice helps increase the nutrient density of your meals. Whole grains can include barley, brown rice, bulgur, oats, rye, and wheat. These grains will help you feel full longer, and their phytochemicals can help fight off disease.

Make beans and legumes a regular part of your diet. Beans and legumes are an excellent source of protein and fiber and have been shown to reduce cholesterol. For example, a staple in the Mediterranean diet is hummus, which is made from chickpeas. Hummus can be eaten with cut-up raw vegetables, such as celery or carrots, and it makes a great afternoon snack. Aim to eat at least ½ cup of beans or legumes daily as a complete part of your diet.

Choose nuts and seeds or nut butters to satisfy a salty snack craving. Nuts and seeds include monounsaturated fats and proteins that not only add beneficial nutrients to your diet, but also increase satiety. When snacking on these options, you will decrease carbohydrate intake and avoid cravings later in the day. Try to eat at least one snack per day that includes nuts or seeds to reduce your risk of heart disease.

Incorporate herbs and spices instead of salt to improve flavors. Herbs and spices can be a tasty way to increase flavor and decrease sodium in the diet. Garlic, for example, is an excellent replacement for added salt and is low in calories, rich in vitamins, and can boost immune health. Limiting your sodium intake to no more than 2,000–2,300 mg per day is an easy way to reduce the risk of hypertension or high blood pressure. For reference, 1 teaspoon of table salt has about 2,300 mg of sodium. Simply adding spices and herbs can substitute for the flavor of salt.

Increase intake of fish and fish oils. As discussed previously, fish oil includes healthy fats and omega-3 fatty acids that decrease inflammation and have been found to reduce the risk of heart disease and arthritis. It is recommended to include 3 to 6 ounces of fish at least twice per week as part of the Mediterranean diet for a healthy dose of these powerful ingredients.

Consume moderate portions of poultry. Chicken is a great source of lean protein. Aim for about one chicken breast (about 3 ounces) two to three times per week to increase your protein intake and decrease your intake of red meat. Avoid frying, and instead bake or grill to avoid unhealthy fats from oils.

Add eggs in moderation. For several years, eggs were considered a contributor to high cholesterol and heart disease. However, recent research has discovered that eggs, when consumed in moderation, can increase essential nutrients such as protein and vitamins and pose no risk to heart health if included as part of a healthy diet. Limit yolk intake to four times per week and use egg whites for other meals as a nutrient-dense protein source. Whole eggs are a complete protein, meaning they include all the essential amino acids, and they increase satiety.

Choose low-fat cheese, milk, and yogurt. Dairy products are a great source of protein, vitamins, and minerals. Milk is fortified with vitamins A and D and packed with calcium to improve bone health. Cheese is loaded with protein and can improve satiety and reduce cravings. Yogurt has healthy bacteria to improve digestive health. Include 6 to 8 ounces of low-fat dairy products three to four times per week to reap all of these benefits while limiting fat intake.

Decrease intake of red meat. Although there are several famous dishes from the Mediterranean that include beef and lamb, these staples are not commonly included in the daily diet. Lamb kebabs and kofta are great for a holiday or family dinner but should be limited to no more than once per week. When choosing ground meats, look for the leanest options and avoid frying to decrease saturated fat intake and promote a healthy cardiovascular system.

Keep the red wine to a minimum. Believe it or not, a glass of wine is permitted in moderation when on the Mediterranean diet. If a small amount (about 5 ounces) is consumed with a meal, it may offer some positive heart effects. The antioxidants in the wine can prevent the buildup of fat in the arteries. Men are permitted 10 ounces daily while women are permitted 5 ounces daily.

Simple Food Swaps

With just a few quick food switches, you can be eating more Mediterranean diet–friendly meals and start reaping the benefits. Some of the food swaps listed here will provide you with healthier options when you're on the go or eating at your favorite restaurant, while others will help with your meal planning at home.

- For your coffee run, order espresso instead of a sugary coffee drink.
- Use herbs and spices for seasoning and marinating dishes instead of sugary sauces and marinades.
- Replace mayonnaise with mashed avocado.
- For happy hour, drink a glass of red wine instead of beer or margaritas.
- For your grab-and-go snack, pack nuts instead of chips.
- Use salmon in place of beef.
- For dessert, enjoy fresh fruit instead of cookies.
- For sandwiches, use whole-grain bread instead of white bread.
- Use olive oil and balsamic vinaigrette in place of processed salad dressings.
- Dip veggies in hummus instead of ranch dressing.

PLATING IT ALL TOGETHER

Here is an example of what a typical Mediterranean diet should look like, with a breakdown of food groups and recommended servings and portion sizes.

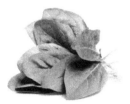

Veggies:
5 servings per day. One serving = 1 cup of raw leafy vegetables, ½ cup of cooked fresh or frozen vegetables, or ½ cup of vegetable juice

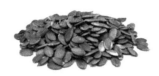

Nuts and seeds:
1 to 2 servings per day. One serving = 2 tablespoons of sunflower seeds, 1 tablespoon of peanut butter or other nut butter, 7 or 8 walnuts or pecans, or 12 to 15 almonds

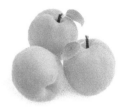

Fruits:
4 to 5 servings per day. One serving = ½ cup of fresh or frozen fruit or ¼ cup of dried fruit or fruit juice

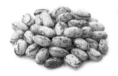

Beans and legumes:
1 to 2 servings per day. One serving = ½ cup of cooked beans or legumes

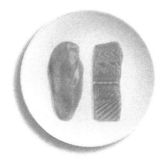

Lean animal proteins:
1 to 3 servings of lean poultry/meat and 2 to 3 servings of fish per week. One serving = 3 ounces (about the size of a deck of cards)

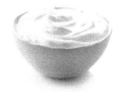

Low-fat dairy products:
1 to 3 servings per day. One serving = 1 cup of low-fat milk or low-fat yogurt or 1½ ounces of cheese (about the size of 6 stacked dice)

Healthy fats:
4 to 6 servings per day. One serving = 1 teaspoon of olive oil, 1 tablespoon of regular salad dressing, ⅛ of an avocado, or 5 olives

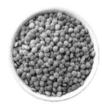

Whole grains:
4 to 6 servings per day. One serving = 1 slice of bread or ½ cup of cooked grains, cereal, or pasta

LIVING THE MEDITERRANEAN LIFE

The Mediterranean "diet" is so much more than just the foods you eat. There are various lifestyle changes that are the keys to succeeding in stress reduction and improved mental and physical health. The lifestyle of the Mediterranean is much more relaxed than in the West, and walking is much more common than driving as a means of transportation. The constant physical activity, at least 30 minutes per day, can help decrease cholesterol, blood sugar, and weight in general.

Even after a hectic work or school day, families head home to prepare and share a meal together and discuss the events of their day. They visit with neighbors or get together for a game of cards in the evening. Weekends are typically spent tending to the fields or gardens, playing outside, or visiting with their friends. A rousing game of soccer may be played at a local court in late afternoon, after the sun's heat has diminished. Cell phones are used to communicate a time to meet or to plan an outing, but otherwise they are put down and conversations happen among family and friends in person. These are some of the many examples of what truly makes up the lifestyle of the Mediterranean.

Here are some realistic suggestions for how you can adopt the Mediterranean lifestyle and decrease the effects of stress on the body. These should not be an afterthought, but rather lifestyle changes that are implemented and planned for, just like planning your next meal.

EATING AND MEALTIMES

Enjoy meals with family and friends. We have a growing tendency to grab a quick meal in our busy lifestyle. In a world of increased stress and decreased free time, try to have at least one meal per day with family and friends. Encourage children to help with meal planning and cooking, divide up tasks such as setting the table or doing dishes, and take time to enjoy the meal with others.

Sit at the dinner table. Studies have shown that sitting down at the table to eat a meal will improve satiety and encourage healthy eating habits. Dinner is the optimal time. Turn off the television and put away the devices. Take the time instead to catch up with those you care about and enjoy a home-cooked meal without distractions.

Eat half of your restaurant meal. There are ways to remain on track with your diet even when eating out. When your meal hits the table, ask the server for a to-go box and place half of your meal inside for the next day. Restaurant portions are usually too large for one person, and this is a great way to cut your calories in half, not feel overly stuffed when you leave, and have a nice treat for another time.

EXERCISE AND RECREATION

Get active after meals. Going for a walk during your lunch break or taking a trip to the park with your kids after brunch on the weekends can encourage a healthy lifestyle for the whole family. Individuals should include 30 minutes of physical activity in the day or aim for 150 minutes per week as part of a heart-healthy diet.

Park a little farther. Anytime we enter the parking lot to our favorite grocery store, most of us skim the spots nearest to the door to see if we are having a lucky day. As part of the Mediterranean lifestyle,

I encourage you to park farther away. After driving for a significant amount of time, it will be good to walk a few extra steps. You may be surprised how many steps you accumulate this way.

Take the stairs. In a world of hectic work days and quick meetings, it is tempting to take the escalator or elevator in order to get to our next stop quickly. However, taking the stairs will add needed physical activity to your day and encourage healthier and sustainable habits to promote physical well-being.

REST AND RELAXATION

Take a break from your phone. You might be wondering how you will keep up with your friends and family without social media, but it is important to detach ourselves from the virtual world to see what is happening in our real world and decrease stress. Have conversations with family members in your home or play a board game together, or meet friends in a park for a walk and catch-up session.

Read a book. Take a walk to your local library and borrow an interesting read. Try to read one to two chapters in the evenings when you're winding down. Not only will this give you some rest and relaxation, but it will help you decrease screen time as well, especially for kids.

Meditate. This form of stress relief is a natural way to retrain your mind, control breathing, and decrease stress and anxiety. Although we may not realize it, anxiety can build subconsciously and impact our health by adding stress to the body and possibly contributing to digestive and heart issues.

WHAT TO EXPECT

Ranked the number one diet overall by *U.S. News & World Report* in 2018 and 2019, the Mediterranean diet can be very attractive. Research has shown its positive effects on blood sugar levels, mood, heart health, weight, and much more. It is important to understand the benefits of the Mediterranean diet and what to expect. These expectations should be managed in order to avoid discouragement if the process of reaching your goals is taking slightly longer than anticipated.

The Mediterranean diet includes some short-term benefits, such as improved mood and enhanced physical fitness. However, there are many long-term benefits, including prevention of chronic disease and treatment of hypertension and high blood sugar. Another long-term effect includes a longer life span. The Mediterranean diet is rich in antioxidants that help combat the aging process, which may be aggravated by stress or pollution.

Although one of the fundamental long-term benefits of this diet is sustainable and maintainable weight loss and weight maintenance, it is important to recognize that this diet is not going to lead to rapid weight loss or a sharp decline in cholesterol levels right off the bat. These goals can be met over time by sustaining improved diet quality and positive lifestyle changes over a longer period of time. It is also important to realize that although weight loss is common when first starting this diet, there may be a plateau that can be overcome by both decreasing portion sizes and increasing physical activity to greater than the recommended daily minimum.

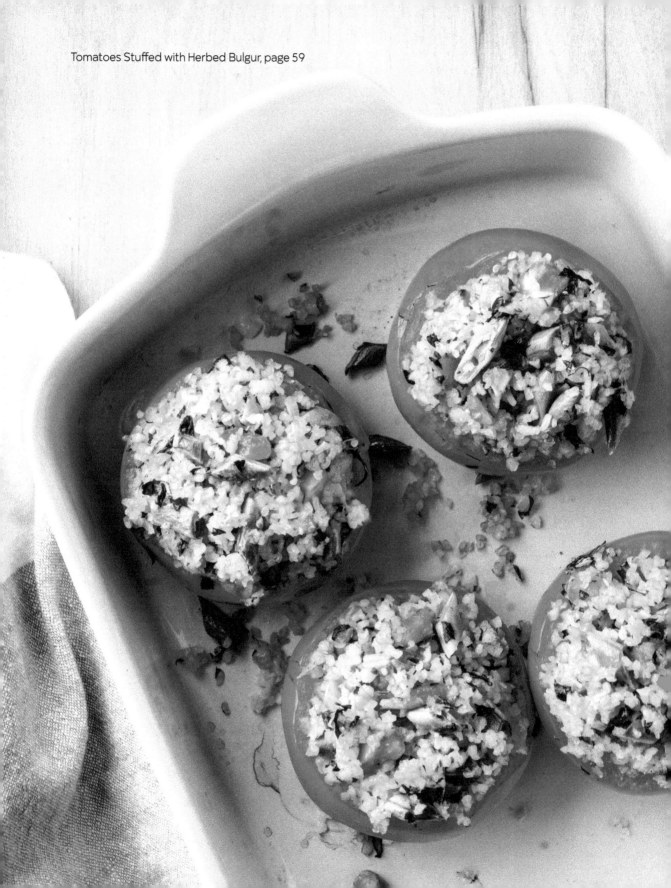
Tomatoes Stuffed with Herbed Bulgur, page 59

CHAPTER 2

The Mediterranean Kitchen and Pantry

A detailed plan is crucial to achieving success with the Mediterranean diet, and part of that plan involves getting your kitchen and pantry ready. Before you embark on the four-week meal plan in part 2, set yourself up with this guide to the essential kitchen equipment and pantry ingredients to make eating healthy easy.

KITCHEN EQUIPMENT AND TOOLS

In order to get cooking Mediterranean style, you will need some equipment and tools to help you along the way. Here is a list of must-have tools to prepare the recipes in this book, as well as a list of nice-to-have (and not terribly expensive) equipment that will make your life so much easier.

MUST-HAVES

Chef's knife: A good knife is the chef's best friend. It is an all-purpose tool for chopping, cutting, slicing, and dicing.

Cutting boards: The partner to the chef's knife, a large cutting board is important in a Mediterranean kitchen.

Silicone spatulas: A silicone spatula is crucial for scraping out the food processor or the sides of the mixing bowl and/or folding eggs when making omelets. Make sure your spatula is silicone and not rubber, or it may melt under high heat.

Tongs: A good pair of tongs keeps your hands at a safe distance from the heat as you toss roasted vegetables and turn chicken or fish fillets. Get a pair that has a durable lock to keep them closed when not in use.

Whisk: Sturdy metal whisks come in all shapes and sizes. Choose a mid-size whisk with a handle that fits comfortably. Use it to mix dry ingredients together before baking, stir eggs for a frittata, or emulsify a vinaigrette.

Measuring cups: It's useful to have a glass measuring cup with ¼-cup, ¾-cup, and 1-cup measurements (or larger for liquid ingredients), as well as individual measuring cups in these same sizes for dry ingredients.

Measuring spoons: A five-piece set will give you a good range for measuring ingredients.

Prep bowls/mixing bowls: This might sound like a no-brainer, but it's important to have a variety of mixing bowls. Get ones that are metal or glass because they're less porous than plastic and they won't pick up stains or odors.

Nonstick skillet: Easy-to-clean, lightweight nonstick pans are ideal for scrambling eggs or wilting greens. Look for ones with ceramic coating, as some nonstick pans are made with PFOAs—chemicals that may be harmful to your health and the environment.

Aluminum baking sheets: Aluminum baking sheets with thick, sturdy rims (rimless baking sheets can lead to burns and spilled food) are perfect for roasting vegetables and other savory stuff.

Set of pots and pans: A large saucepan is essential for making pasta, boiling potatoes, and simmering big batches of soups and broths. Look for a 5- or 6-quart size. A smaller saucepan (1½ or 2½ quarts) comes in handy for smaller items, like boiled eggs, rice, and oatmeal.

Grater: This handy item helps with grating cheese, carrots, apples, cucumbers, and more.

Set of glass or BPA-free plastic storage containers: Storage containers help with organizing your refrigerator and storing leftovers.

NICE-TO-HAVES

Instant-read thermometer: With this handy tool, you can easily check the doneness of your meat and fish.

Food processor: A food processor allows you to blend, chop, dice, and slice with ease for quicker meal preparation.

Immersion blender: This handheld tool makes it so easy to blend soups, smoothies, and pestos with the push of a button. I find it much easier to handle than a traditional blender, and it's great because it takes up much less space.

Timer: Timing is everything when it comes to cooking. If you're making multiple items at once, it's crucial to keep track of individual cooking times.

Garlic press: This small tool is a convenient and time-saving alternative to chopping and gives you uniformly minced garlic without the mess. Simply place a peeled garlic clove in and the press does all the work.

Mandoline: A mandoline is a hand-operated slicing machine with various-size blades that makes thinly slicing firm foods easier and faster. I can slice a whole zucchini, potato, or onion in about 10 seconds.

Kitchen scale: A kitchen scale will help with portion control and may be handy if you are preparing recipes that specify weight (as in baking).

PANTRY STAPLES

Having some key ingredients stocked and ready to use in your pantry will make your success in following the Mediterranean diet easier. Here is a list of Mediterranean staples to get you started, and a few recipes from this book to inspire you to incorporate each one into your diet.

Whole grains: Because whole grains are loaded with nutrients, fiber, and protein, they are considered "good carbs" and an important factor in eating a healthy, balanced diet. Enjoy dishes using whole grains, such as barley, brown rice, bulgur, and quinoa, like Oatmeal Bowls with Blackberries, Seeds, and Honey (page 124) and Citrus-Chicken Vegetable "Risotto" (page 37).

Olive oil: Olives and olive oil are widely used in Mediterranean cuisine. Olive oil is the main source of fat in the Mediterranean diet and is used for cooking, baking, and salad dressings. Try the Kalamata Olive and Sweet Pepper Frittata (page 28) and Couscous-Avocado Salad (page 176).

Dark leafy greens: Dark leafy greens, like collards, spinach, arugula, and kale, are a nutritional power-house. They are a great source of fiber and contain vitamins C and K, as well as iron, calcium, and other antioxidants. Enjoy some of these power greens with the Chicken Shawarma Bowls (page 112) and Sautéed Dark Leafy Greens (page 164).

Garlic: Garlic works in just about anything from salad dressings and marinades to roasted vegetables and stews. You'll get plenty of garlic with my Baking Sheet Spicy Shrimp with Vegetables (page 108) and Egg-Stuffed Portobello Mushrooms (page 129).

Nuts and seeds: Nuts are a great choice for a snack, as they are loaded with protein, fiber, and heart-healthy fats. You can sprinkle sesame or sunflower seeds over a salad or toss them with roasted vegetables for a little added nutrition. You will certainly get your fill of nuts in the Quinoa Nuts and Seeds Overnight Porridge (page 25).

Beans and lentils: Beans are loaded with protein and fiber and are a great alternative to meat. Make quick meals using canned beans, but be sure to rinse the beans before using to remove some of the added sodium. Try the Moroccan Couscous Salad (page 104) or Chickpea Veggie Burgers (page 109) for a hearty meat-free meal.

Eggs: Eggs are a high-quality source of protein and are regularly used in Mediterranean cuisine. The Loaded Smoked Salmon Breakfast Casserole (page 75) and Goat Cheese, Spinach, and Egg Frittata (page 53) are just two of the many delicious recipes incorporating eggs.

Fish: Fish contains heart-healthy omega-3 fatty acids and is widely served in Mediterranean cuisine. Enjoy fish twice weekly. Salmon, sardines, and mackerel are all great choices high in omega-3s. Try the Broiled Flounder with Nectarine and White Bean Salsa (page 142) or Baked Sardine Patties (page 143).

Medjool dates: Medjool dates are the fruits of the date palm tree. Dates can be enjoyed as is, but I find they're very versatile in the kitchen. They can be used to naturally sweeten smoothies, granola bars, and desserts. In this book, you can find dates in the Spiced Oranges with Dates (page 185) and Sweet Kale Smoothie (page 49).

Honey: Honey is among the most versatile foods you can have in your pantry, and cooking with honey will add a whole new dimension to your food. Sweet or savory, healthy or decadent, the natural sweetness of honey adds something very special to a range of dishes and drinks. Enjoy honey with Golden Oatmeal Pancakes (page 27) and Lemon-Spinach Salad with Pears and Blue Cheese (page 101).

SPICE UP YOUR LIFE

Herbs and spices are a cornerstone of Mediterranean cuisine. They are a healthier option than many sauces and seasonings, and brighten up foods without the added fats and calories. Beyond their amazing flavors, many spices and herbs have disease-preventing properties.

Thyme: A popular all-purpose herb, thyme is a native of Southern Europe and a mainstay for flavoring soups, stews, and sauces. It has a delicate taste and does not easily overwhelm other flavors in a dish, making it very versatile in the kitchen. Two recipes in this book that use thyme are Balsamic-Basted Beef Kebabs with Barley and Spinach Risotto (page 33) and Roasted Vegetable Mélange (page 175).

Cumin: Cumin is sold both ground and as whole seeds. The strongly aromatic spice is popular in North African cuisine, as well as South Asian dishes. For added flavor, toast the whole seeds before use. You will be able to taste this delicious spice in the Salmon Bowl with Bulgur and Tahini Sauce (page 85) and Halibut with Olive-Tomato Sauce (page 87).

Rethinking Your Freezer

Your freezer is an amazing appliance, and if you stock it with the right foods, you'll not only eat better, but you'll stress less, too, because you'll know you have all the components to make a great meal waiting for you. Here are a few things to keep in your freezer:

Frozen fruits and vegetables: These are flash frozen at peak ripeness and are as nutrient-rich as fresh produce, making them the perfect solution during months that fresh produce just isn't available.

Pre-prepped smoothie ingredients: Having freezer bags with prepped, individually portioned smoothie ingredients makes it that much easier to make a healthy choice for breakfast or a snack. Make a bunch of these and enjoy them all month long.

Veggie scraps: Keep a bag in the freezer at all times to store veggie scraps. Any time you chop an onion, peel a carrot, or have any leftover bits and pieces from aromatic veggies, add them to the bag. When it's full, use it to make homemade veggie stock. It's so much better than the store-bought kind and is a great ingredient to have on hand for cooking risottos, sautéing greens, and, of course, making soup.

Fresh herbs: Let's be honest. Most of us buy fresh herbs and never end up using them all. Instead of letting them rot in the back of your refrigerator, freeze them for later use. Hardier herbs like rosemary, thyme, and sage can be frozen in a single layer on a plate and stored in an airtight freezer bag, whereas leafier herbs like basil, mint, and cilantro can be chopped up, mixed with olive oil, and frozen in ice cube trays to flavor soups and stews and make salad dressings.

Go nuts! Nuts are cheaper when bought in bulk. Stick them in the freezer so they don't go rancid so fast.

Oregano: Commonly used in Greek, Spanish, and Italian cuisine, oregano is a perennial herb and relative of mint. Greek and Spanish oregano have the strongest flavor of the three varieties. Oregano is found in a number of recipes in this book, like the Turkey-Tomato Ragù (page 154) and Greek Herbed Beef Meatballs (page 161).

Coriander: Coriander is often used in Spanish, Mexican, Latin, and Indian cuisine, and works particularly well with onions, bell peppers, tomatoes, and potatoes. Enjoy lots of coriander in the Moroccan Spiced Chicken with Sweet Potato Hash (page 88) and Moroccan Couscous Salad (page 104).

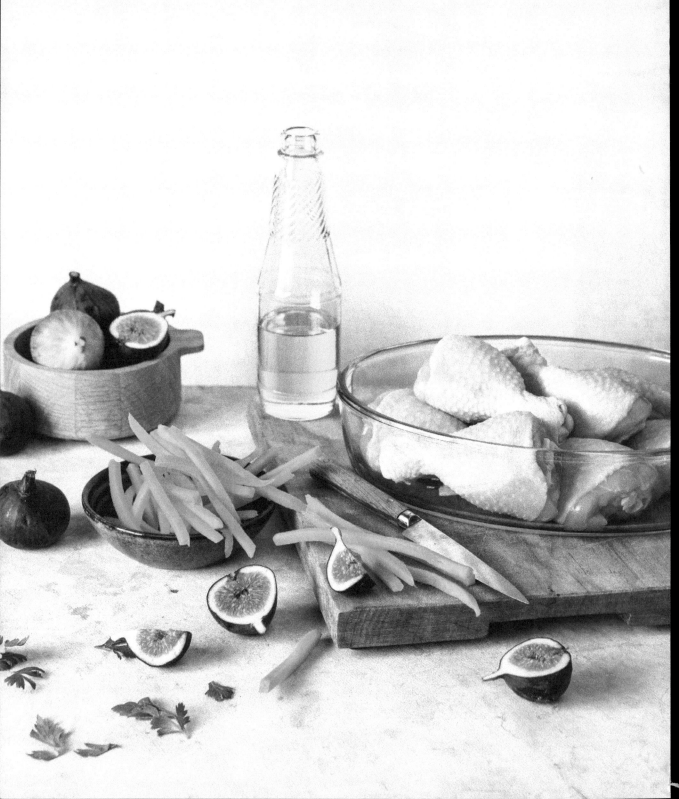

PART TWO

WEEKLY MEAL PLAN

WITH RECIPES

Hurray! You are officially on your way to starting a healthier diet and lifestyle. Before you dive in, let's take a quick look at the elements of each chapter and how to use them. Each chapter includes a meal plan, which lays out what you will be eating for the week. You can rearrange the meals as needed to fit your schedule. You'll also find a couple of simple snack ideas for each week, a handy shopping list you can snap a photo of to take with you to the store, and a prep guide for preparing ingredients and dishes ahead of time. Store prepped ingredients in sealed containers in the refrigerator until ready to use. The recipes for each week are included right in the chapter for your convenience. Most are written to serve four to six people, but the meal plan is structured for two, so there will be plenty of leftovers to enjoy throughout the week.

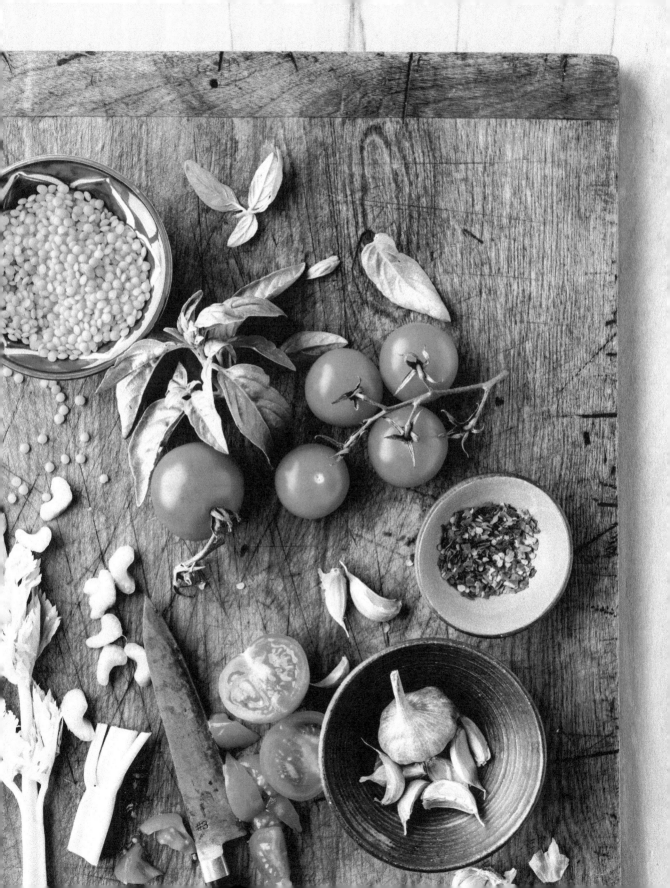

CHAPTER 3

Week One
Meal Plan and Recipes

Welcome to your first week of the Mediterranean diet! This is a very exciting week, and you have a lot of fun and delicious recipes to look forward to. If you've never had quinoa before, you are in for a treat, as it's used in a couple of recipes this week and it's one of my favorite grains. At first, it may seem daunting to get all your shopping done, prep for the week ahead, and cook homemade meals every day, but before you know it, you'll be an expert. I promise you, each week will get easier, and your confidence level will build.

WEEK ONE MEAL PLAN

	BREAKFAST	LUNCH	DINNER
MON	Quinoa Nuts and Seeds Overnight Porridge* (page 25)	Quinoa and Spinach Salad with Figs and Balsamic Dressing (page 30)	Balsamic-Basted Beef Kebabs with Barley and Spinach Risotto* (page 33)
TUE	*Leftover* Quinoa Nuts and Seeds Overnight Porridge	*Leftover* Balsamic-Basted Beef Kebabs with Barley and Spinach Risotto	Tomato and Lentil Soup* (page 35)
WED	Low-fat Greek yogurt and berries	Green Vegetable Wrap with Basil Pesto (page 31)	Halibut with Wilted Kale and Cherry Tomatoes (page 36)
THU	Chia-Pomegranate Smoothie (page 26)	*Leftover* Tomato and Lentil Soup	Citrus-Chicken Vegetable "Risotto"* (page 37)
FRI	Low-fat Greek yogurt and berries	*Leftover* Citrus-Chicken Vegetable "Risotto"	Simple Bouillabaisse* (page 39)
SAT	Golden Oatmeal Pancakes (page 27)	*Leftover* Simple Bouillabaisse	Shaved Cucumber Quinoa Bowl (page 41)
SUN	Kalamata Olive and Sweet Pepper Frittata* (page 28)	Grilled Vegetable Open-Faced Sandwich (page 32)	Lemon-Garlic Skillet Chicken* (page 42)

*These dishes will be eaten later in the week as leftovers, so make extra if needed.

WEEK ONE SNACK IDEAS

CELERY AND ALMOND BUTTER: Celery and almond butter are the perfect pair for curbing your appetite. Spread 1 tablespoon of almond butter on a couple stalks of celery.

AVOCADO ON MULTIGRAIN CRACKERS: Mash 1 peeled and seeded avocado with the juice of ½ lime and salt and pepper to taste. Spread about 1 tablespoon on a few multigrain crackers.

WEEK ONE SHOPPING LIST

Canned and Bottled Items

- Almond milk, vanilla, unsweetened (½ cup)
- Balsamic dressing (½ cup)
- Lentils, red, low-sodium (1 [15-ounce] can)
- Pesto, basil (¼ cup)
- Pomegranate juice (1 cup)
- Stock, chicken, low-sodium (3 cups)
- Stock, fish (4 cups)
- Stock, vegetable, low-sodium (6 cups)
- Tomatoes, diced, low-sodium (2 [28-ounce] cans)
- Tomatoes, sun-dried, oil-packed (½ cup)

Dairy and Eggs

- Cheese, cottage, low-fat (8 ounces)
- Cheese, feta (2 ounces)
- Cheese, goat (4 ounces)
- Cheese, Parmesan, grated (1 ounce)
- Eggs, large (13)
- Milk, low-fat (½ cup)

Frozen

- Berries, mixed (1 cup)

Meat

- Beef, top sirloin steak (1 pound)
- Chicken, breast tenders, boneless, skinless (1 pound)
- Chicken, rotisserie (2 cups)
- Halibut (4 [4-ounce] fillets)
- Mussels (10)
- Salmon, flounder, or halibut fillets (12 ounces)
- Shrimp, large (10)

Pantry Items

- Barley, pearled
- Bay leaf
- Black pepper, ground
- Chia seeds
- Cinnamon, ground
- Coriander, ground
- Cumin, ground
- Dates, Medjool
- Honey
- Mustard, Dijon
- Oats, rolled, gluten-free
- Oil, coconut
- Oil, olive
- Pecans
- Pine nuts
- Pumpkin seeds
- Quinoa
- Red pepper flakes
- Rice, brown
- Sea salt
- Sunflower seeds
- Vanilla extract
- Vinegar, balsamic
- Vinegar, white wine

Produce

- Basil (1 bunch)
- Bell pepper, green (1)
- Bell peppers, red (3)
- Bell pepper, yellow (1)
- Broccoli (1 small head)
- Carrot (1)
- Cauliflower (1 small head)
- Celery (1 bunch)
- Cucumbers, English (3)
- Eggplant, small (1)
- Fennel (1 bulb)
- Figs (8)
- Garlic (2 heads)
- Green beans (16)
- Kale (1 bunch)
- Lemons (6)
- Onions, sweet (3)
- Onions (2)
- Oregano (1 bunch)
- Parsley (1 bunch)
- Scallions (1 bunch)
- Spinach (18 ounces)
- Thyme (1 bunch)
- Tomatoes (4)
- Tomatoes, cherry (1 pint)
- Tomatoes, plum (2)
- Zucchini, small (1)

Other

- Bread, Italian or French (4 slices)
- Olives, green, pitted (½ cup)
- Olives, Kalamata, pitted (½ cup)
- Tortillas, whole-wheat (4)

WEEK ONE OPTIONAL PREP GUIDE

Wash and Cut

- Cauliflower: finely chop 1 cup
- Fennel: chop
- Green beans: trim
- Green bell pepper: slice
- Kale: wash and chop
- Red bell pepper: chop 2
- Spinach: wash and dry all, thinly slice 1 cup, chop 10 cups
- Yellow bell pepper: finely chop

Cook and Store

- Quinoa: 2 cups
- Vegetables (zucchini, eggplant, onion, 1 red bell pepper): grill

Make Ahead

- Quinoa Nuts and Seeds Overnight Porridge (page 25)
- Tomato and Lentil Soup (page 35)

WEEK ONE RECIPE LIST

- Quinoa Nuts and Seeds Overnight Porridge
- Chia-Pomegranate Smoothie
- Golden Oatmeal Pancakes
- Kalamata Olive and Sweet Pepper Frittata
- Quinoa and Spinach Salad with Figs and Balsamic Dressing
- Green Vegetable Wrap with Basil Pesto
- Grilled Vegetable Open-Faced Sandwich
- Balsamic-Basted Beef Kebabs with Barley and Spinach Risotto
- Tomato and Lentil Soup
- Halibut with Wilted Kale and Cherry Tomatoes
- Citrus-Chicken Vegetable "Risotto"
- Simple Bouillabaisse
- Shaved Cucumber Quinoa Bowl
- Lemon-Garlic Skillet Chicken

Quinoa Nuts and Seeds Overnight Porridge

SERVES 4 • DAIRY-FREE • GLUTEN-FREE • MEAL IN ONE • VEGETARIAN

PREP TIME:
10 MINUTES, PLUS
COOLING TIME

COOK TIME:
15 MINUTES

Overnight oats are one of the easiest preparations to start the day on a healthy note. Crunchy seeds and nuts and a drizzle of sweet honey dress it up. Soaking oats improves their digestibility because their phytic acid is reduced and the starches in the oats break down. After cooked oats are cooled, their digestion-resistant starch increases, helping you feel full longer.

½ cup quinoa

1 cup water

1 cup gluten-free rolled oats

½ cup unsweetened vanilla almond milk, plus more if needed

¼ cup pumpkin seeds

¼ cup chopped pecans

1 tablespoon honey

1. Rinse the quinoa under cold running water to remove its bitter flavor. In a small saucepan, combine the quinoa and water and bring to a boil over medium heat. Reduce the heat to low and simmer, uncovered, until the liquid is absorbed, 10 to 15 minutes. Set aside to cool.

2. In a medium bowl, stir together the cooled quinoa, oats, almond milk, pumpkin seeds, pecans, and honey until well mixed. Transfer to a storage container and store in the refrigerator, sealed, overnight.

3. Stir in more almond milk in the morning if needed to adjust the texture. Serve.

COOKING TIP: *Cooked quinoa will last up to 1 week in the refrigerator or for 8 months in the freezer, so it is simple to whip up a large batch to use for many recipes. Make sure you use cooked quinoa because raw quinoa has a bitter taste and can cause stomach upset.*

PER SERVING: *Calories: 282; Total fat: 9g; Saturated fat: 1g; Carbohydrates: 42g; Sugar: 5g; Fiber: 5g; Protein: 10g*

Chia-Pomegranate Smoothie

SERVES 2 • DAIRY-FREE • GLUTEN-FREE • MEAL IN ONE • VEGAN • 30 MINUTES OR LESS

PREP TIME:
5 MINUTES

Pomegranate is considered one of the first cultivated fruits and a symbol of fertility in many cultures. This distinctive fruit adds color and a tangy flavor to this smoothie as well as a significant nutritional impact. Pomegranate contains three times more antioxidants than berries or green tea and is an excellent source of vitamin C, fiber, and vitamin K. Regularly including pomegranate in your diet can boost your immune system and decrease the risk of cardiovascular disease and several types of cancer.

1 cup pure pomegranate juice (no sugar added)

1 cup frozen berries

1 cup coarsely chopped kale

2 tablespoons chia seeds

3 Medjool dates, pitted and coarsely chopped

Pinch ground cinnamon

In a blender, combine the pomegranate juice, berries, kale, chia seeds, dates, and cinnamon and pulse until smooth. Pour into glasses and serve.

INGREDIENT TIP: *Medjool dates are wonderful, but other dates can be used if they are difficult to find. You can also order them online both pitted and with pits.*

PER SERVING: *Calories: 275; Total fat: 5g; Saturated fat: 1g; Carbohydrates: 59g; Sugar: 10g; Fiber: 42g; Protein: 5g*

Golden Oatmeal Pancakes

SERVES 4 • GLUTEN-FREE • MEAL IN ONE • VEGETARIAN • 30 MINUTES OR LESS

PREP TIME:
5 MINUTES

COOK TIME:
20 MINUTES

Pancakes seem like a guilty pleasure—almost like eating cake for breakfast. What about pancakes made with wholesome oats and low-fat cottage cheese, and flavored with vanilla and a hint of sweet honey? You can even top them with fresh fruit and a drizzle of maple syrup and still start your day off right. Cinnamon adds a lovely spicy taste and is known to have blood sugar–lowering properties, including reducing insulin resistance. This warm spice and the addition of oats can help stabilize your blood sugar all day.

4 large egg whites

1 large egg

1 cup low-fat cottage cheese

2 tablespoons honey

1 teaspoon vanilla extract

½ teaspoon ground cinnamon

1 cup gluten-free rolled oats

Coconut oil, for cooking

1. In a large bowl, whisk together the egg whites, egg, cottage cheese, honey, vanilla, and cinnamon until well blended and most of the lumps are gone. Whisk in the rolled oats until blended.

2. Place a large skillet over medium heat and lightly coat it with coconut oil.

3. Pour about ¼ cup of batter onto the skillet for each pancake, being sure not to overcrowd. Cook until the tops of the pancakes start to bubble, about 3 minutes, then flip the pancakes. Cook until the other side is golden brown, about 2 more minutes. Repeat with the rest of the batter. Serve warm or cold.

COOKING TIP: *Cold pancakes are a perfect snack with a little nut butter or wrapped around fresh fruit. Double the batch, cool the extras, and store in the refrigerator wrapped in plastic for up to 3 days.*

PER SERVING: *Calories: 164; Total fat: 3g; Saturated fat: 1g; Carbohydrates: 19g; Sugar: 9g; Fiber: 1g; Protein: 15g*

Kalamata Olive and Sweet Pepper Frittata

SERVES 4 • GLUTEN-FREE • MEAL IN ONE • VEGETARIAN • 30 MINUTES OR LESS

PREP TIME:
10 MINUTES

COOK TIME:
15 MINUTES

The word "frittata" conjures mornings lounging on sunny Italian patios enjoying a delicious breakfast and stunning vistas. Much more romantic than a plain omelet, this beauty is bursting with gorgeous roasted peppers, olives, and creamy goat cheese. Oregano is an herb people often associate with Italian cuisine, and the most common type used in Italy is Sicilian oregano, which is rich in disease-fighting and inflammation-reducing antioxidants.

1 tablespoon olive oil

1 sweet onion, chopped

1 red bell pepper, chopped

1 teaspoon minced garlic

8 large eggs

½ cup low-fat milk

½ cup pitted, sliced Kalamata olives

¼ cup chopped fresh oregano

½ cup crumbled goat cheese

Sea salt

Freshly ground black pepper

1. Preheat the oven to broil.

2. In a large ovenproof skillet, heat the olive oil over medium heat. Sauté the onion, bell pepper, and garlic until softened, about 4 minutes.

3. In a small bowl, whisk together the eggs, milk, olives, and oregano until well blended. Pour the egg mixture into the skillet and as the mixture starts to set, lift the edges with a spatula, and let the egg flow under the cooked portions.

4. Continue cooking and lifting until the egg mixture is almost set, 5 to 7 minutes.

5. Sprinkle the top of the frittata with goat cheese and place the entire skillet in the oven.

6. Broil until the eggs are set and the top is golden brown, about 2 minutes. Season with salt and pepper and serve.

COOKING TIP: *For a different preparation, divide the sautéed vegetables and egg mixture evenly between 8 muffin cups and bake until almost set in a 375°F oven, about 20 minutes. Increase the heat to broil, top the muffins with the goat cheese, and broil for about 2 minutes.*

PER SERVING: *Calories: 287; Total fat: 19g; Saturated fat: 7g; Carbohydrates: 12g; Sugar: 5g; Fiber: 4g; Protein: 18g*

Quinoa and Spinach Salad with Figs and Balsamic Dressing

SERVES 4 • GLUTEN-FREE • MEAL IN ONE • VEGETARIAN

PREP TIME:
10 MINUTES, PLUS
COOLING TIME

COOK TIME:
15 MINUTES

Figs and balsamic vinegar pair beautifully: sweet and sour in perfect balance. Figs are very perishable, so use them in this pretty salad within a couple of days of buying them. This fruit is packed with potassium, iron, magnesium, calcium, and vitamin B_6; it improves digestion and reduces the risk of hypertension and bad cholesterol, as well as lowers blood sugar. For a weekday lunch, cook the quinoa the night before and assemble the rest of the salad when you're ready to eat.

½ cup quinoa

1 cup water

6 cups chopped spinach

8 ripe figs, quartered

¼ cup sunflower seeds

½ cup store-bought balsamic dressing

½ cup crumbled goat cheese

1. Rinse the quinoa under cold running water to remove its bitter flavor. In a small saucepan, combine the quinoa and water and bring to a boil over medium heat. Reduce the heat to low and simmer, uncovered, until the liquid is absorbed, 10 to 15 minutes. Transfer to a dish and refrigerate until cool.

2. In a large bowl, toss the spinach, cooled quinoa, figs, and sunflower seeds until well mixed. Add the dressing, toss to coat, and transfer the salad to serving plates. Top with goat cheese and serve.

SUBSTITUTION TIP: *For a dairy-free and vegan option, leave out the goat cheese topping. Or you can find good-quality vegan cheese options at most grocery stores.*

PER SERVING: *Calories: 348; Total fat: 12g; Saturated fat: 3g; Carbohydrates: 54g; Sugar: 21g; Fiber: 7g; Protein: 11g*

Green Vegetable Wrap with Basil Pesto

SERVES 4 • MEAL IN ONE • VEGETARIAN • 30 MINUTES OR LESS

PREP TIME:
15 MINUTES

When cut, wraps can look like works of art. The different shades of green vegetables plus the creamy white feta cheese create a lovely spring-like palette on your plate. Green beans are high in fiber, protein, iron, vitamins C and K, and carotenoids such as beta-carotene, lutein, and chlorophyll. Green beans reduce the risk of most chronic diseases like cancer, cardiovascular disease, and diabetes.

¼ cup store-bought or homemade basil pesto

4 whole-wheat tortillas

1 cup shredded spinach

1 green bell pepper, cut into thin strips

½ English cucumber, cut into ¼-inch batons

16 green beans, trimmed

1 scallion, both white and green parts, thinly sliced on the bias

¼ cup crumbled feta cheese

1. Spread the pesto on the tortillas, about 1 tablespoon each, to about 1 inch from the edge.

2. Layer with the spinach, bell pepper, cucumber, green beans, and scallion in the center of each tortilla and sprinkle with feta cheese.

3. Fold the sides of the first tortilla in toward the center over the vegetables, and then roll from the end closest to you, tucking the tortilla and filling in as you roll. Repeat with the remaining tortillas and serve.

COOKING TIP: *You can make your own pesto by puréeing 2 cups of fresh basil leaves, ½ cup of Parmesan cheese, ¼ cup of pine nuts, and 1 tablespoon of minced garlic in a food processor; with the motor running, add ½ cup of olive oil in a thin stream until well combined. Store in a sealed container in the refrigerator for up to 2 weeks.*

PER SERVING: *Calories: 318; Total fat: 18g; Saturated fat: 3g; Carbohydrates: 37g; Sugar: 6g; Fiber: 10g; Protein: 9g*

Grilled Vegetable Open-Faced Sandwich

SERVES 4 • MEAL IN ONE • VEGETARIAN

PREP TIME:
15 MINUTES

COOK TIME:
21 MINUTES

This colorful sandwich will be messy eating with piles of vegetables and a generous splash of balsamic vinegar, so don't forget your napkins. The combination of peppers and tomatoes ensures a healthy dose of disease-fighting antioxidants, such as lycopene, beta-carotene, and quercetin. Adding eggplant to the mix can help protect against cardiovascular disease and neurological issues.

3 cups sliced vegetables (eggplant, zucchini, onion, and red bell pepper)

2 tablespoons olive oil, divided

4 (1-inch-thick) slices crusty Italian or French bread

½ cup sliced sun-dried tomatoes

¼ cup crumbled feta cheese

1 tablespoon balsamic vinegar

2 tablespoons chopped fresh oregano, for garnish

1. Preheat the oven to 450°F.

2. In a large bowl, toss the vegetables and 1 tablespoon of olive oil and arrange on a baking sheet. Cook for 20 minutes, stirring once about halfway through, until tender.

3. Preheat the broiler.

4. Brush both sides of the bread with the remaining 1 tablespoon of olive oil and broil, turning once, until the bread is golden, about 1 minute total.

5. Evenly divide the sun-dried tomatoes between the toast slices and top with an assortment of the grilled vegetables. Divide the feta cheese between the sandwiches and drizzle with balsamic vinegar. Garnish with oregano and serve.

COOKING TIP: *You can also make quesadillas using whole-grain tortillas instead of bread. Broil the tortillas for 30 seconds on each side after brushing them with olive oil or grill them on a barbecue until crisp and lightly charred.*

PER SERVING: *Calories: 297; Total fat: 7g; Saturated fat: 2g; Carbohydrates: 48g; Sugar: 9g; Fiber: 5g; Protein: 11g*

Balsamic-Basted Beef Kebabs with Barley and Spinach Risotto

SERVES 4 • DAIRY-FREE • MEAL IN ONE

PREP TIME:
15 MINUTES, PLUS
MARINATING TIME

COOK TIME:
55 MINUTES

This is a complete meal, perfect for company or a special family barbecue. Spinach is a crucial component both visually and for its earthy taste. Spinach first makes an appearance in Mediterranean writings over 1,000 years ago and remains a commonly used ingredient in many cuisines in the area. Called a superfood, it is incredibly rich in iron, lutein, protein, and vitamins A, C, and E, as well as folic acid, calcium, and potassium. Including this dark leafy green in your diet regularly will reduce your risk of high blood pressure, cancer, and macular degeneration.

¼ cup olive oil, divided

2 tablespoons balsamic vinegar

2 teaspoons Dijon mustard

1 pound beef top sirloin steak, cut into 1-inch cubes

½ sweet onion, finely chopped

1 red bell pepper, chopped

2 teaspoons minced garlic

1 cup pearled barley, rinsed

3 cups low-sodium chicken stock

4 cups chopped spinach

2 tablespoons pine nuts

1 tablespoon chopped fresh thyme

Sea salt

1. In a large bowl, stir together 3 tablespoons of olive oil, balsamic vinegar, and mustard until blended. Add the beef to the bowl, toss to coat, cover, and refrigerate for 30 minutes. Soak bamboo skewers in warm water.

2. While the meat is marinating, in a large saucepan, heat the remaining 1 tablespoon of olive oil over medium-high heat. Sauté the onion, bell pepper, and garlic until softened, about 4 minutes.

Continued >

Balsamic-Basted Beef Kebabs with Barley and Spinach Risotto

Continued

3. Stir in the barley and chicken stock and bring to a boil. Reduce the heat to low, cover, and simmer until the barley is tender and the liquid is absorbed, about 40 minutes.

4. Remove from the heat and stir in the spinach, pine nuts, and thyme. Season with salt.

5. Preheat a grill to medium high.

6. Thread the beef onto the soaked wooden skewers, leaving space between each chunk.

7. Grill the skewers until the beef reaches desired doneness, turning occasionally, about 10 minutes total for medium. Serve the beef skewers on the barley risotto.

SUBSTITUTION TIP: *The best vinegar to use for this marinade is an aged balsamic because it adds depth of flavor, but other products will do in a pinch. Regular balsamic, apple cider vinegar, champagne vinegar, and red wine vinegar are distinctive and pair well with red meat. If you do not have a grill, broil the kebabs in the oven for 8 to 10 minutes total, turning once.*

PER SERVING: *Calories: 445; Total fat: 15g; Saturated fat: 1g; Carbohydrates: 45g; Sugar: 3g; Fiber: 10g; Protein: 33g*

Tomato and Lentil Soup

SERVES 4 • DAIRY-FREE • GLUTEN-FREE • MEAL IN ONE • VEGAN

PREP TIME:
10 MINUTES

COOK TIME:
35 MINUTES

Tomato soup gets a bad rap because of all the bland versions from a can. This homemade version captures all the goodness and flavor of summer in a bowl. If you have access to fresh tomatoes in season, try using those instead of canned. The lentils add a healthy dose of protein and vitamin B_6.

1 tablespoon olive oil

1 sweet onion, chopped

2 celery stalks, chopped

1 tablespoon minced garlic

6 cups low-sodium vegetable stock

2 (28-ounce) cans low-sodium diced tomatoes

1 (15-ounce) can low-sodium red lentils, rinsed and drained

1 tablespoon chopped fresh basil

Pinch red pepper flakes

Sea salt

Freshly ground black pepper

1. In a large pot, heat the olive oil over medium-high heat. Sauté the onion, celery, and garlic until softened, about 3 minutes.

2. Stir in the stock and tomatoes with their juices and bring to a boil. Reduce the heat to low and simmer for 20 minutes.

3. In a food processor, purée the soup until smooth. Return the soup to the pot and stir in the lentils, basil, and red pepper flakes and simmer until heated through, about 10 minutes. Season with salt and pepper and serve.

PER SERVING: *Calories: 211; Total fat: 4g; Saturated fat: 1g; Carbohydrates: 36g; Sugar: 11g; Fiber: 13g; Protein: 12g*

Halibut with Wilted Kale and Cherry Tomatoes

SERVES 4 • DAIRY-FREE • GLUTEN-FREE • MEAL IN ONE • 30 MINUTES OR LESS

PREP TIME:
10 MINUTES

COOK TIME:
15 MINUTES

f your schedule is tight but you still want a nutritious, delicious meal, look no further than this flaky white fish nestled in healthy greens and vibrant tomatoes! Combining the kale and lemon is a good idea because the vitamin C in lemon makes the iron in kale more easily absorbed by the body.

2 tablespoons olive oil, divided

3 cups coarsely chopped kale

2 cups halved cherry tomatoes

4 (4-ounce) boneless, skinless halibut fillets

Juice and zest of 1 lemon

Sea salt

Freshly ground black pepper

1 tablespoon chopped fresh basil

1. Preheat the oven to 375°F. Lightly grease an 8-by-8-inch baking dish with 2 teaspoons of olive oil.

2. Arrange the kale in the bottom of the baking dish and top with the cherry tomatoes and the halibut. Drizzle the remaining 1 tablespoon plus 1 teaspoon of olive oil and the lemon juice over the dish and season with salt and pepper. Sprinkle with lemon zest and basil.

3. Bake until the fish flakes easily and the greens are wilted, about 15 minutes. Serve.

COOKING TIP: *You can also cook the fish and vegetables in individual foil packets on a baking sheet instead of in a baking dish for easy serving. Just divide the ingredients evenly between 4 (12-by-12-inch) sheets of foil, fold them up into tight bundles, and bake for the same time.*

PER SERVING: *Calories: 228; Total fat: 10g; Saturated fat: 2g; Carbohydrates: 9g; Sugar: 2g; Fiber: 2g; Protein: 28g*

Citrus-Chicken Vegetable "Risotto"

SERVES 4 • GLUTEN-FREE • MEAL IN ONE

PREP TIME:
25 MINUTES, PLUS
COOLING TIME

COOK TIME:
30 MINUTES

You will not have to stand over a saucepan spooning hot broth and endlessly stirring to create this tempting risotto because it is created with cold-cooked rice instead. The simple Parmesan dressing adds richness and that cheesy accent so loved in traditional risotto. You can toss the dressing into the hot rice before chilling to produce an almost creamy texture. Parmesan cheese is an excellent source of protein, the most protein-dense cheese of all, and is easily digestible due to its aging process.

FOR THE DRESSING

Juice and zest of 1 lemon

½ teaspoon minced garlic

¼ cup olive oil

¼ cup grated Parmesan cheese

Sea salt

Freshly ground black pepper

FOR THE RISOTTO

1 cup brown rice, soaked overnight and drained

1½ cups water

2 cups chopped store-bought rotisserie chicken or leftover cooked chicken

1 cup finely chopped cauliflower

1 yellow bell pepper, finely chopped

1 carrot, finely chopped

2 tomatoes, seeded and chopped

1 scallion, both white and green parts, thinly sliced

2 tablespoons chopped fresh oregano

TO MAKE THE DRESSING

In a small bowl, whisk together the lemon juice, lemon zest, garlic, olive oil, and Parmesan cheese. Season with salt and pepper and set aside.

Continued >

Citrus-Chicken Vegetable "Risotto"

Continued

TO MAKE THE RISOTTO

1. In a large pot, combine the soaked rice and water. Bring to a boil, reduce the heat to low, cover, and simmer for 20 to 30 minutes, until tender. Transfer to a dish and refrigerate until cool.

2. In a large bowl, mix together the cooled rice, chicken, cauliflower, bell pepper, carrot, tomatoes, scallion, and oregano. Stir in the dressing and toss to combine. Serve.

COOKING TIP: *Brown rice can take a long time to cook. Cut down on this time by soaking the rice over-night (or for at least 8 hours) in the refrigerator in a 1:2 rice-to-water ratio. If you don't soak the rice, increase the cooking time to 45 minutes, and use 2 cups of water.*

PER SERVING: *Calories: 330; Total fat: 16g; Saturated fat: 3g; Carbohydrates: 25g; Sugar: 5g; Fiber: 4g; Protein: 24g*

Simple Bouillabaisse

SERVES 4 • DAIRY-FREE • GLUTEN-FREE • MEAL IN ONE

PREP TIME:
10 MINUTES

COOK TIME:
35 MINUTES

Bouillabaisse is a classic French stew originating in the southern region of France, probably in Marseille. Fresh seafood is the base of this dish along with delicate fennel-flavored broth. Don't forget to save the feathery fennel fronds to use as a pretty garnish or in another recipe. Many of the nutrients from the fennel bulb, such as potassium, vitamins A and C, and calcium, are also present in the tops.

1 tablespoon olive oil

½ sweet onion, chopped

3 celery stalks, chopped

1 cup chopped fennel

1 tablespoon minced garlic

4 cups fish stock or clam juice

2 tomatoes, chopped

1 tablespoon chopped fresh thyme

1 bay leaf

¼ teaspoon red pepper flakes

10 mussels, scrubbed and debearded

12 ounces boneless, skinless fish fillets, cut into 1-inch chunks (salmon, flounder, or halibut)

10 large shrimp, peeled and deveined

1 cup shredded kale

Sea salt

Freshly ground black pepper

1. In a large, deep skillet, heat the olive oil over medium-high heat. Sauté the onion, celery, fennel, and garlic until softened, about 6 minutes.

2. Add the fish stock, tomatoes, thyme, bay leaf, and red pepper flakes and bring to a boil. Reduce the heat to low and simmer for 10 minutes.

Continued >

Simple Bouillabaisse

Continued

3. Add the mussels, cover the skillet, and simmer for 2 minutes more.

4. Add the fish and shrimp, cover, and simmer until the mussels open and the fish is just cooked through, 8 to 10 minutes.

5. Discard the bay leaf and add the kale to the skillet. Cover and remove from the heat and let stand for 5 minutes so the kale wilts. Season with salt and pepper and serve immediately.

SUBSTITUTION TIP: *The joy of bouillabaisse is that any type of seafood will work. Mussels can be fresh or frozen, in the shell or just the meat. You can throw in clams instead of mussels, as well. If you use canned clams, add the juice for extra flavor.*

PER SERVING: *Calories: 353; Total fat: 20g; Saturated fat: 5g; Carbohydrates: 12g; Sugar: 3g; Fiber: 3g; Protein: 31g*

Shaved Cucumber Quinoa Bowl

SERVES 4 • DAIRY-FREE • GLUTEN-FREE • MEAL IN ONE • VEGAN

PREP TIME:
15 MINUTES, PLUS
COOLING TIME

COOK TIME:
15 MINUTES

You will be delighted by how pretty these wide cucumber ribbons look on the plate and how easy they are to create. Cucumbers are a stellar source of vitamins A, C, and K, as well as potassium and calcium.

1 cup quinoa

2 cups water

2 English cucumbers

2 plum tomatoes, cut into eighths

1 cup chopped broccoli

½ cup pitted, sliced green olives

1 scallion, both white and green parts, chopped

1 tablespoon chopped fresh oregano

¼ cup olive oil

2 tablespoons white wine vinegar

Sea salt

Freshly ground black pepper

1. Rinse the quinoa under cold running water to remove its bitter flavor. In a small saucepan, combine the quinoa and water and bring to a boil over medium heat. Reduce the heat to low and simmer, uncovered, until the liquid is absorbed, 10 to 15 minutes. Transfer to a dish and refrigerate until cool.

2. While the quinoa is cooking, use a vegetable peeler to shave the cucumbers into long strips. Arrange the cucumbers on a large platter.

3. In a large bowl, stir together the cooled quinoa, tomatoes, broccoli, olives, scallion, and oregano. Spoon the quinoa mixture into the center of the cucumber noodles.

4. In a small bowl, whisk together the olive oil and vinegar and season with salt and pepper. Drizzle the dressing over the entire dish and serve.

PER SERVING: *Calories: 358; Total fat: 18g; Saturated fat: 3g; Carbohydrates: 43g; Sugar: 8g; Fiber: 7g; Protein: 10g*

Lemon-Garlic Skillet Chicken

SERVES 4 • DAIRY-FREE • GLUTEN-FREE

PREP TIME:
10 MINUTES, PLUS
MARINATING TIME

COOK TIME:
15 MINUTES

This simple one-skillet meal is perfect for a busy weeknight. Plan a little extra time to marinate the chicken in advance, and you can be ready to eat in 15 minutes. Not only do lemons so brightly season simple meals like this, they also are an excellent source of vitamin C and are high in potassium and vitamin B_1.

¼ cup freshly squeezed lemon juice

4 tablespoons olive oil, divided

6 garlic cloves, minced

1 tablespoon chopped fresh oregano

1 teaspoon ground cumin

1 teaspoon ground coriander

1 pound boneless, skinless chicken breast tenders

Sea salt

Freshly ground black pepper

1 onion, sliced

2 lemons, cut into wedges

Chopped fresh parsley, for garnish

1. In a medium bowl, combine the lemon juice, 2 tablespoons of olive oil, garlic, oregano, cumin, and coriander and mix well.

2. Season the chicken with salt and pepper and then place the chicken and the onion in the marinade. Toss to coat. Cover and let rest for at least 20 minutes or refrigerate for up to 8 hours.

3. In a large cast iron skillet, heat the remaining 2 tablespoons of olive oil over medium heat.

4. Add the chicken tenders to the skillet in a single layer, discarding any marinade left behind.

5. Cook on each side for 6 to 7 minutes, flipping once, until browned and the juices run clear.

6. Transfer the chicken and onions to a serving platter. Serve with the lemon wedges and garnish with parsley.

SUBSTITUTION TIP: *Replace the chicken breast tenders with boneless, skinless chicken thighs if desired. Or if you have chicken breasts on hand, simply prepare them for this recipe by cutting each breast into four or five lengthwise strips.*

PER SERVING: *Calories: 349; Total fat: 21g; Saturated fat: 3g; Carbohydrates: 7g; Sugar: 3g; Fiber: 2g; Protein: 40g*

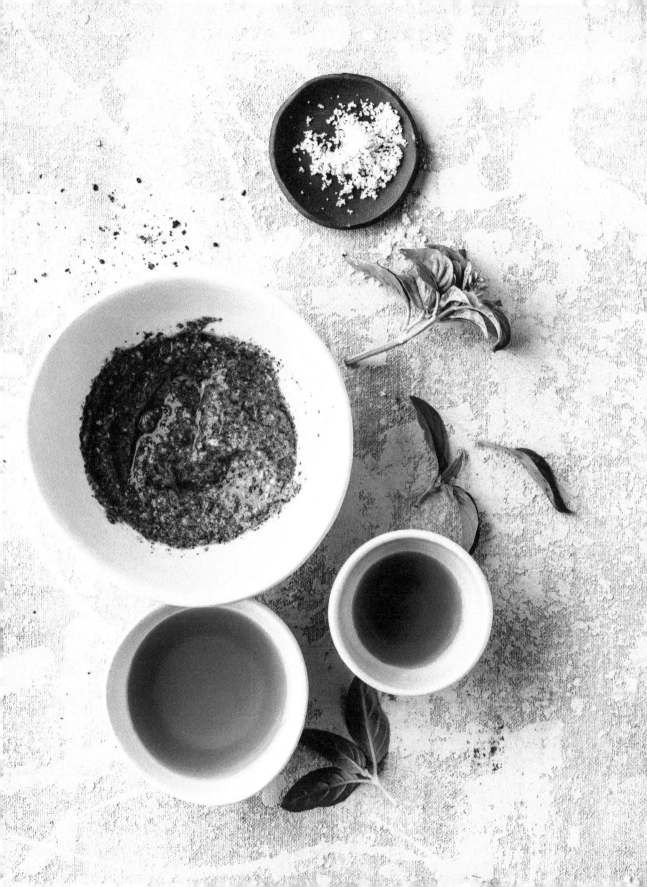

CHAPTER 4

Week Two
Meal Plan and Recipes

You've conquered week one, which is probably the most difficult week of all, so pat yourself on the back for a job well done. In week two, you'll really start getting the hang of things, and your confidence level should creep up as a result. There are many wonderful recipes to enjoy this week. The Sweet Kale Smoothie (page 49) is one of my favorites. Kale is considered a superfood, and for good reason: It's loaded with anti-oxidants, nutrients, and digestive support. By the end of the week, you should be feeling more energetic, and a little lighter, too.

WEEK TWO MEAL PLAN

	BREAKFAST	LUNCH	DINNER
MON	*Leftover* Kalamata Olive and Sweet Pepper Frittata (from Week 1)	*Leftover* Lemon-Garlic Skillet Chicken (from Week 1)	Oven-Roasted Puttanesca with Ground Beef* (page 56)
TUE	Sweet Kale Smoothie (page 49)	*Leftover* Oven-Roasted Puttanesca with Ground Beef	Citrus-Artichoke Pesto with Vegetable Noodles* (page 58)
WED	Multigrain toast with avocado; an apple	*Leftover* Citrus-Artichoke Pesto with Vegetable Noodles	Tomatoes Stuffed with Herbed Bulgur* (page 59)
THU	Savory Hummus Breakfast Toasts (page 50)	*Leftover* Tomatoes Stuffed with Herbed Bulgur	Tuna Couscous Bowl with Grilled Vegetables* (page 61)
FRI	Sweet Kale Smoothie (page 49)	*Leftover* Tuna Couscous Bowl with Grilled Vegetables	Trout with Roasted Red Pepper Sauce (page 63)
SAT	Asparagus, Apple, and Feta Cheese Omelet (page 51)	Salmon, Citrus, and Avocado Salad (page 54)	Greek Roasted Vegetable Bowl (page 64)
SUN	Goat Cheese, Spinach, and Egg Frittata* (page 53)	Sun-dried Tomato and Olive Tapenade with Goat Cheese Toasts (page 55)	Chicken with Yogurt-Mint Sauce (page 65)

*These dishes will be eaten later as leftovers, so make extra if needed.

WEEK TWO SNACK IDEAS

CARROTS AND HUMMUS: Since you're going to be making hummus anyway, make some extra for a snack this week. A handful of carrots with 3 tablespoons of hummus makes a good-size portion.

HARD-BOILED EGGS: Make plenty of this protein-licious snack in advance to munch on any time of the day. Enjoy by itself and/or with 1 or 2 multigrain crackers or 1 slice of whole-grain toast.

WEEK TWO SHOPPING LIST

Canned and Bottled Items

- Anchovies 1 (4-ounce) can
- Apple juice (½ cup)
- Artichoke hearts, marinated (2 [12-ounce] jars)
- Capers (1 teaspoon)
- Chickpeas (2 [15-ounce] cans)
- Pesto, basil (2 tablespoons)
- Roasted red peppers (2 [12-ounce] jars)
- Salmon, boneless, skinless (2 [5-ounce] cans)
- Tomatoes, sun-dried, oil-packed (2 [10-ounce] jars)
- Tuna, water-packed (2 [5-ounce] cans)

Dairy and Eggs

- Cheese, Asiago, shredded (1 ounce)
- Cheese, feta, crumbled (3 ounces)
- Cheese, goat, crumbled (4 ounces)
- Cheese, Parmesan, grated (½ ounce)
- Eggs, large (16)
- Milk, low-fat (¼ cup)
- Yogurt, plain, low-fat, Greek (2 cups)

Meat

- Beef, ground, extra-lean (8 ounces)
- Chicken, breast, boneless, skinless (4 [3-ounce] fillets)
- Trout (4 [4-ounce] fillets)

Pantry Items

- Black pepper, ground
- Bulgur
- Couscous
- Cumin, ground
- Dates, Medjool
- Fettucine, whole-grain, dry
- Oil, olive
- Pecans, halved
- Pine nuts
- Red pepper flakes
- Sea salt
- Tahini
- Vinegar, apple cider

Produce

- Apples (2)
- Asparagus (1 bunch)
- Avocado (1)
- Basil (1 bunch)
- Bell pepper, red (1)
- Bell pepper, yellow (1)
- Butternut squash (1)
- Carrots (3)
- Celery root (1)
- Cucumber, English (1)
- Dill (1 bunch)
- Eggplant, small (1)
- Garlic (2 heads)
- Grapefruits, ruby red (2)
- Green beans (10 ounces)
- Greens, mixed baby (12 ounces)
- Kale (6 ounces)
- Lemons (7)
- Mint (1 bunch)
- Onion, red (1)
- Onions, sweet (3)
- Oranges (2)
- Oregano (1 bunch)
- Parsley (1 bunch)

- Parsnips (2)
- Scallion (1)
- Spinach (8 ounces)
- Tomatoes (12)
- Zucchini, green, large (4)

Other

- Baguette, whole-grain (1)
- Bread, multigrain (4 slices)
- Olives, Kalamata, pitted (2 cups)

WEEK TWO OPTIONAL PREP GUIDE

Wash and Cut

- Asparagus: chop
- Baby mixed greens: wash and dry
- Butternut squash: peel and chop into 1-inch pieces
- Carrots: peel and chop 2 into 1-inch pieces, store in water
- Kale: wash and dry, coarsely chop
- Parsnips: peel and chop into 1-inch pieces, store in water
- Red bell pepper: slice into 1-inch strips
- Spinach: wash and dry all, chop 1 cup, shred 1 cup, store remaining leaves whole
- Yellow bell pepper: slice into 1-inch strips
- Zucchini: spiralize 3 large

Cook and Store

- Bulgur: 1 cup

Make Ahead

- Pesto Vinaigrette (page 190)

WEEK TWO RECIPE LIST

- Sweet Kale Smoothie
- Savory Hummus Breakfast Toasts
- Asparagus, Apple, and Feta Cheese Omelet
- Goat Cheese, Spinach, and Egg Frittata
- Salmon, Citrus, and Avocado Salad
- Sun-dried Tomato and Olive Tapenade with Goat Cheese Toasts
- Oven-Roasted Puttanesca with Ground Beef
- Citrus-Artichoke Pesto with Vegetable Noodles
- Tomatoes Stuffed with Herbed Bulgur
- Tuna Couscous Bowl with Grilled Vegetables
- Trout with Roasted Red Pepper Sauce
- Greek Roasted Vegetable Bowl
- Chicken with Yogurt-Mint Sauce

Sweet Kale Smoothie

SERVES 2 • GLUTEN-FREE • MEAL IN ONE • VEGETARIAN • 30 MINUTES OR LESS

PREP TIME:
10 MINUTES

Smoothies seem like a logical choice on the Mediterranean diet because healthy vegetables and fruit are the cornerstones of this lifestyle and this blended drink. Kale combines extremely well with other ingredients, especially fresh lemon juice, which brightens the flavor of this nutrient-packed dark leafy green. Kale's health benefits come from high levels of vitamins and minerals (vitamins A, B, and C; calcium, potassium, and magnesium) and phytonutrients (beta-carotene, alpha-linoleic acid, and chlorophyll). Kale can support the digestive system, increase testosterone, promote healthy eyesight, and reduce the risk of heart disease and type 2 diabetes.

1 cup low-fat plain Greek yogurt

½ cup apple juice

1 apple, cored and quartered

4 Medjool dates

3 cups packed coarsely chopped kale

Juice of ½ lemon

4 ice cubes

1. In a blender, combine the yogurt, apple juice, apple, and dates and pulse until smooth.

2. Add the kale and lemon juice and pulse until blended. Add the ice cubes and blend until smooth and thick. Pour into glasses and serve.

INGREDIENT TIP: *If you are not a regular kale eater, it might be best to reduce the amount of this green to about 1 cup and replace the other 2 cups with spinach. Large amounts of raw kale can cause bloating and stomach issues if you are not used to it.*

PER SERVING: *Calories: 355; Total fat: 2g; Saturated fat: 1g; Carbohydrates: 77g; Sugar: 58g; Fiber: 8g; Protein: 11g*

Savory Hummus Breakfast Toasts

SERVES 4 • MEAL IN ONE • VEGETARIAN • 30 MINUTES OR LESS

PREP TIME:
10 MINUTES

COOK TIME:
3 MINUTES

Instead of sugar-packed jam and peanut butter on your toast, try a savory version in the morning. The toppings piled on this hummus toast can be anything, but some ingredients will boost the health benefits of the meal. Carrots and hummus provide protein, healthy fat, and fiber. In addition, vitamin A from the carrots helps the body synthesize the protein and magnesium in the chickpeas and increases the absorption of magnesium, so the process that releases fat from its stores in the body (lipolysis) is also accelerated.

4 multigrain bread slices

½ cup Traditional Hummus (page 188) or store-bought hummus

½ cup sliced English cucumber

½ cup shredded carrot

¼ cup chopped oil-packed sun-dried tomatoes

1 scallion, both white and green parts, thinly sliced on the bias

¼ cup crumbled feta cheese

2 tablespoons sliced Kalamata olives

1. Toast the bread and spread 2 tablespoons of hummus on each slice.

2. Divide the cucumber, carrot, sun-dried tomatoes, scallion, feta cheese, and olives between the toasts. Serve.

INGREDIENT TIP: *Sun-dried tomatoes can also be purchased dried in bags. If you are using the dried product, be sure to reconstitute the tomatoes first by soaking them in water before chopping.*

PER SERVING: *Calories: 166; Total fat: 7g; Saturated fat: 2g; Carbohydrates: 20g; Sugar: 4g; Fiber: 5g; Protein: 8g*

Asparagus, Apple, and Feta Cheese Omelet

SERVES 4 • GLUTEN-FREE • MEAL IN ONE • VEGETARIAN

PREP TIME:
20 MINUTES

COOK TIME:
20 MINUTES

This satisfying omelet is one of my favorites to make for breakfast. It is also great for an easy lunch or dinner, or you can serve it on a bed of greens for a heartier meal. Asparagus is loaded with glutathione, a powerful antioxidant, and is a good source of protein, potassium, and vitamins A, C, K, and B_6. Paired with eggs, apple, and spinach, this nutrient-dense omelet will keep you feeling full longer.

2 tablespoons olive oil, divided

8 asparagus spears, chopped

1 garlic clove, minced

1 cup chopped spinach

¼ cup peeled chopped apple

1 tablespoon chopped fresh oregano

1 tablespoon chopped fresh basil

Sea salt

¼ cup chopped roasted red peppers

6 large eggs

¼ cup low-fat milk

⅓ cup crumbled feta cheese

1. In a large skillet, heat 1 tablespoon of olive oil over medium heat. Cook the asparagus, stirring, for 4 to 5 minutes, until softened. Add the garlic and cook for 1 minute.

2. Add the spinach, apple, oregano, and basil. Season lightly with salt and continue cooking until the apples are softened and spinach has cooked down, about 5 minutes. Stir in the roasted red peppers and transfer the vegetables to a plate.

3. In a small bowl, whisk the eggs with the milk.

Continued >

Asparagus, Apple, and Feta Cheese Omelet

Continued

4. Wipe out the skillet, then heat the remaining 1 tablespoon of olive oil over medium heat and pour the eggs into the pan. As the eggs firm up, lift the edges and let the uncooked egg flow underneath, cooking until the eggs are almost set but still moist, 7 to 8 minutes. Season with salt.

5. Spoon the vegetable mixture onto one side of the omelet and sprinkle with the feta cheese. Fold the other half of the omelet over the cheese mixture and cook for 1 to 2 minutes more. Cut into slices and serve.

SUBSTITUTION TIP: *Omelets are so versatile. If you don't have the recipe ingredients on hand, or simply want to try a different flavor profile, you can substitute any ingredients you like. Try arugula or baby kale instead of the spinach, pear instead of the apple, and crumbled goat cheese or shredded mozzarella instead of the feta.*

PER SERVING: *Calories: 369; Total fat: 31g; Saturated fat: 12g; Carbohydrates: 7g; Sugar: 5g; Fiber: 2g; Protein: 17g*

Goat Cheese, Spinach, and Egg Frittata

SERVES 4 • GLUTEN-FREE • MEAL IN ONE • VEGETARIAN • 30 MINUTES OR LESS

PREP TIME:
10 MINUTES

COOK TIME:
15 MINUTES

Tangy, rich goat cheese is very high in calcium, and eggs are an excellent source of vitamin D. Calcium is not easily absorbed by the body unless paired with vitamin D, so this frittata is well planned as well as delicious.

1 tablespoon olive oil

2 cups spinach

1 sweet onion, chopped

1 teaspoon minced garlic

5 large eggs

5 large egg whites

Sea salt

Freshly ground black pepper

½ cup coarsely chopped roasted red peppers

½ cup crumbled goat cheese

1 tablespoon chopped fresh parsley

1. Preheat the oven to broil.

2. In a large ovenproof skillet, heat the olive oil over medium-low heat and sauté the spinach, onion, and garlic until softened, about 5 minutes.

3. Whisk together the eggs and egg whites and season lightly with salt and pepper. Pour the eggs into the skillet. As they firm up, lift the edges with a spatula and let the uncooked egg flow underneath. Cook until eggs are almost set, 7 to 8 minutes.

4. Scatter the roasted red peppers and goat cheese over the top of the frittata and broil until the top is completely set and the cheese is melted, 1 to 2 minutes. Serve topped with parsley.

PER SERVING: *Calories: 213; Total fat: 14g; Saturated fat: 6g; Carbohydrates: 5g; Sugar: 3g; Fiber: 1g; Protein: 17g*

Salmon, Citrus, and Avocado Salad

SERVES 4 • DAIRY-FREE • GLUTEN-FREE • MEAL IN ONE • 30 MINUTES OR LESS

PREP TIME:
20 MINUTES

Salad is a quick meal choice that does not always have to be light. This salad is satisfying and energy boosting. Avocado is very rich in the monounsaturated fat that staves hunger, so the low-calorie base leafy greens don't seem unsubstantial. Salmon is also rich in healthy fats and vitamin D, which, when combined with the magnesium in the greens, can significantly reduce the risk of colon cancer and cardiovascular disease.

6 cups mixed baby greens (spinach, kale, and Swiss chard)

2 large oranges, peeled, segmented, and cut into chunks

2 ruby red grapefruits, peeled, segmented, and cut into chunks

1 avocado, peeled, pitted, and chopped

2 (5-ounce) cans boneless, skinless salmon, drained

½ cup pecan halves

½ cup Pesto Vinaigrette (page 190)

1. Arrange the greens on a large platter and top with the oranges, grapefruits, avocado, salmon, and pecans.

2. Drizzle the salad with the vinaigrette and serve.

SUBSTITUTION TIP: *Pecans are a tree nut, so they can be an allergen for many people. If this is an issue for you, swap them out for sunflower or pumpkin seeds, in the same amount, to add a satisfying crunch.*

PER SERVING: *Calories: 459; Total fat: 34g; Saturated fat: 5g; Carbohydrates: 28g; Sugar: 13g; Fiber: 8g; Protein: 19g*

Sun-dried Tomato and Olive Tapenade with Goat Cheese Toasts

SERVES 4 • MEAL IN ONE • 30 MINUTES OR LESS

PREP TIME:
20 MINUTES

COOK TIME:
5 MINUTES

This rich tapenade is sublime when topped with sweet sun-dried tomatoes and creamy goat cheese. Goat's milk cheese is a great source of calcium, amino acids, protein, iron, and vitamins A, B, C, and D.

1 cup pitted Kalamata olives

3 anchovy fillets

2 garlic cloves, peeled

1 teaspoon capers

2 tablespoons olive oil

1 tablespoon freshly squeezed lemon juice

Pinch red pepper flakes

2 tablespoons chopped fresh parsley

1 whole-grain baguette, cut on the bias into 8 (1-inch-thick) slices

1 cup chopped oil-packed sun-dried tomatoes

½ cup crumbled goat cheese

1. Preheat the oven to broil.

2. In the food processor, combine the olives, anchovies, garlic, capers, olive oil, lemon juice, red pepper flakes, and parsley and pulse until the ingredients are finely chopped.

3. Place the bread on a baking sheet and broil until toasted on both sides, turning once, about 2 minutes total.

4. Spread 1 tablespoon of tapenade on each piece of bread and evenly divide the sun-dried tomatoes between the bread slices.

5. Sprinkle with goat cheese and broil until the cheese is melted, about 1 minute. Serve.

PER SERVING: *Calories: 364; Total fat: 17g; Saturated fat: 5g; Carbohydrates: 40g; Sugar: 5g; Fiber: 4g; Protein: 15g*

Oven-Roasted Puttanesca with Ground Beef

SERVES 4 • MEAL IN ONE

PREP TIME:
10 MINUTES

COOK TIME:
35 MINUTES

This recipe is inspired by the traditional puttanesca invented in Naples. You will be boosting the incredible tomato flavor by roasting this ingredient and adding the intensity of sun-dried tomatoes. Whole-grain pasta offers twice as much fiber as regular pasta to support a healthy bowel. Whole-grain pasta is also high in B vitamins, which help make red blood cells, support nerve health, repair DNA, and are crucial for turning your food into energy.

6 large tomatoes (about 2 pounds), cut into wedges

1 sweet onion, coarsely chopped

½ cup chopped sun-dried tomatoes

4 garlic cloves, thinly sliced

2 tablespoons olive oil, divided

8 ounces whole-grain fettucine

8 ounces extra-lean ground beef

½ cup pitted, halved Kalamata olives

¼ cup shredded fresh basil

Pinch red pepper flakes

Sea salt

Freshly ground black pepper

2 tablespoons grated Parmesan cheese

1. Preheat the oven to 425°F and line a baking sheet with aluminum foil.

2. In a medium bowl, combine the tomatoes, onion, sun-dried tomatoes, garlic, and 1 tablespoon of olive oil and toss well. Transfer the tomato mixture to the baking sheet and roast in the oven until very tender, about 30 minutes.

3. While the vegetables are roasting, bring a large pot of water to a boil and cook the pasta according to package instructions until al dente. Drain.

4. While the pasta is cooking, in a large saucepan, add the remaining 1 tablespoon of olive oil and heat over medium-high heat. Brown the ground beef, about 10 minutes. Remove any oil from the pot with a spoon and discard.

5. Add the roasted vegetables to the saucepan along with the olives, basil, and red pepper flakes and stir to combine well, breaking up any larger chunks of vegetables.

6. Stir in the pasta. Season with salt and pepper and serve topped with Parmesan cheese.

SUBSTITUTION TIP: *If you want a vegetarian option or a lighter meal, this sauce is equally delicious without the ground beef. Leave out the Parmesan cheese topping as well to make the dish vegan.*

PER SERVING: *Calories: 433; Total fat: 15g; Saturated fat: 3g; Carbohydrates: 56g; Sugar: 13g; Fiber: 7g; Protein: 23g*

Citrus-Artichoke Pesto with Vegetable Noodles

SERVES 4 • GLUTEN-FREE • MEAL IN ONE • VEGETARIAN • 30 MINUTES OR LESS

PREP TIME:
25 MINUTES

This dish of fresh vegetable noodles topped with fragrant pesto delights the senses and evokes bright spring days. If you don't have a spiralizer, you can use a vegetable peeler to create lengthwise flat noodles.

2 cups chopped marinated artichoke hearts, divided

½ cup packed fresh basil leaves

½ cup pine nuts

1 tablespoon minced garlic

Zest and juice from 1 lemon

¼ cup olive oil

Sea salt

Freshly ground black pepper

3 large green zucchinis, spiralized

Pinch red pepper flakes

¼ cup shredded Asiago cheese

1. In a food processor, place 1 cup of artichoke hearts, basil, pine nuts, garlic, lemon zest, lemon juice, and olive oil and pulse until very finely chopped and a thick paste forms. Season with salt and pepper.

2. In a large bowl, toss the zucchini noodles, remaining 1 cup of artichoke hearts, and red pepper flakes until well mixed.

3. Add the pesto 1 tablespoon at a time until you have the desired flavor. Serve the vegetable noodles immediately topped with Asiago cheese. Store any leftover pesto in a sealed container in the refrigerator for up to 2 weeks.

PER SERVING: *Calories: 350; Total fat: 31g; Saturated fat: 5g; Carbohydrates: 15g; Sugar: 6g; Fiber: 5g; Protein: 8g*

Tomatoes Stuffed with Herbed Bulgur

SERVES 4 • DAIRY-FREE • VEGAN

PREP TIME:
10 MINUTES

COOK TIME:
40 MINUTES

Because this preparation is so easy and versatile, stuffed vegetables can be found in many Mediterranean countries, such as France, Spain, Greece, and Italy. Almost any ingredients can be combined and spooned into tomatoes, so use your imagination. This combination is effective because green beans and tomatoes create optimal iron absorption to boost muscle and brain health. Iron is crucial for the production of hemoglobin, which is the mode of transport for oxygen throughout the body.

1 cup bulgur

2 cups water

4 large tomatoes

1 tablespoon olive oil

½ sweet onion, finely chopped

2 teaspoons minced garlic

2 cups green beans, cut into ½-inch pieces

2 tablespoons chopped fresh parsley

1 tablespoon chopped fresh basil

1 tablespoon chopped fresh oregano

Juice and zest of 1 lemon

Sea salt

Freshly ground black pepper

1. In a small pot, combine the bulgur and water. Bring to a boil, cover, and reduce the heat to simmer and cook until tender, about 15 minutes. Drain any extra water and set aside.

2. Preheat the oven to 400°F.

3. Cut the tops off the tomatoes and scoop out the pulp and seeds with a spoon. Place the tomato shells, cut-side up, into a 9-by-9-inch baking dish and set aside. Chop the pulp and seeds coarsely, and transfer to a bowl.

Continued >

Tomatoes Stuffed with Herbed Bulgur

Continued

4. In a medium skillet, heat the olive oil. Sauté the onion and garlic until softened, about 3 minutes. Stir in the tomato pulp, green beans, parsley, basil, oregano, lemon juice, and lemon zest. Sauté for 1 minute and remove from the heat.

5. Stir in the cooked bulgur and toss to combine. Season with salt and pepper. Spoon the bulgur mixture into the tomatoes and bake until the tomatoes are very soft, about 20 minutes. Serve.

SUBSTITUTION TIP: *Stuffed vegetables are incredibly versatile, so they can be prepared to suit any diet or allergy issue. If gluten is a concern, try black beans, lentils, quinoa, or even riced cauliflower in place of the bulgur.*

PER SERVING: *Calories: 197; Total fat: 5g; Saturated fat: 1g; Carbohydrates: 36g; Sugar: 6g; Fiber: 10g; Protein: 6g*

Tuna Couscous Bowl with Grilled Vegetables

SERVES 4 • DAIRY-FREE • MEAL IN ONE

PREP TIME:
20 MINUTES

COOK TIME:
15 MINUTES

This filling salad is a combination of several types of cuisines, from the North African couscous to Greek grilled vegetables and Italian parsley. Parsley is one of the most popular herbs in Italian cooking and is one of the most nutritious herbs you can eat, even if it is often found as a garnish in restaurants. Packed with chlorophyll, beta-carotene, iron, and vitamins A, C, and K, parsley can boost the immune system, purify the blood, and reduce the risk of atherosclerosis, stroke, cancer, and diabetes.

1½ cups water

1 cup couscous

½ small eggplant, cut into ¼-inch slices

1 red bell pepper, cut into 1-inch strips

1 yellow bell pepper, cut into 1-inch strips

1 large zucchini, cut lengthwise into ¼-inch strips

½ red onion, cut into ¼-inch slices

1 tablespoon olive oil

Sea salt

Freshly ground black pepper

2 (5-ounce) cans water-packed tuna, drained

2 tomatoes, cut into wedges

¼ cup chopped fresh parsley

Juice from 1 lemon

1. In a pot, bring the water to a boil. Stir in the couscous, remove from the heat, cover, and let sit for 10 minutes. Fluff with a fork.

2. In a medium bowl, toss the eggplant, bell peppers, zucchini, onion, and olive oil and season with salt and pepper.

3. Preheat a grill to medium-high heat.

Continued >

Tuna Couscous Bowl with Grilled Vegetables

Continued

4. Grill the vegetables until they are lightly charred and softened, turning once, about 6 minutes total. Transfer the vegetables to a plate to cool for 10 minutes. Chop the vegetables into 1-inch chunks.

5. Evenly divide the couscous between bowls and arrange the grilled vegetables, tuna, and tomatoes on top. Sprinkle with parsley and squeeze the lemon juice over each bowl. Serve.

COOKING TIP: *If you do not have a grill, the vegetables can be prepared on baking sheets in a 450°F oven. Coat them with the olive oil, salt, and pepper and spread them on a baking sheet. Roast in the oven, turning once, until tender and lightly browned, 10 to 12 minutes total.*

PER SERVING: *Calories: 354; Total fat: 5g; Saturated fat: 1g; Carbohydrates: 48g; Sugar: 5g; Fiber: 7g; Protein: 30g*

Trout with Roasted Red Pepper Sauce

SERVES 4 • DAIRY-FREE • GLUTEN-FREE • 30 MINUTES OR LESS

PREP TIME:
15 MINUTES

COOK TIME:
6 MINUTES

Simple ingredients cooked so that their flavors and textures shine through is one of the goals of cooking. Lightly seasoned pan-fried flaky trout topped with bright, rich pepper sauce meets that criterion. Look for deep red bell peppers because the deeper the color, the higher the concentration of antioxidants. Bell peppers are very high in vitamins A, B, C, and E, calcium, potassium, and zinc. This combination of nutrients detoxes the body, boosts the immune system, lowers cholesterol, and helps prevent cardiovascular disease.

2 cups store-bought or homemade roasted red peppers

1 teaspoon minced garlic

Juice of 1 lemon

4 (4-ounce) trout fillets

Sea salt

Freshly ground black pepper

1 tablespoon olive oil

2 tablespoons chopped fresh parsley

1. In a blender, combine the roasted red peppers, garlic, and lemon juice and pulse until smooth. Set aside.

2. Lightly season the trout with salt and pepper.

3. In a large skillet, heat the olive oil over medium-high heat. Cook the fillets for about 3 minutes, then flip and cook until the fish is just cooked through and lightly golden, about 3 minutes. Serve topped with a generous spoonful of roasted red pepper sauce and a sprinkle of parsley.

COOKING TIP: *To roast your own peppers, lightly coat them with olive oil and roast on a baking sheet in a 450°F oven until lightly charred all over, about 25 minutes. Place them in a bowl and cover with plastic wrap until the skins loosen and you can peel them easily.*

PER SERVING: *Calories: 229; Total fat: 12g; Saturated fat: 3g; Carbohydrates: 7g; Sugar: 3g; Fiber: 0g; Protein: 23g*

Greek Roasted Vegetable Bowl

SERVES 4 • DAIRY-FREE • GLUTEN-FREE • MEAL IN ONE • VEGAN

PREP TIME:
15 MINUTES

COOK TIME:
40 MINUTES

Roasted root vegetables, lightly caramelized, make an ideal base for a satisfying bowl. Butternut squash adds brilliant sunny color to this dish, and boosts the immune system, protects the eyes from age-related decline, and supports bone health.

1 butternut squash, peeled, seeded, and cut into 1-inch chunks

1 celery root, peeled and cut into 1-inch chunks

2 carrots, peeled and cut into 1-inch chunks

2 parsnips, peeled and cut into 1-inch chunks

1 tablespoon olive oil

Sea salt

Freshly ground black pepper

1 cup shredded spinach

½ cup chopped marinated artichoke hearts

¼ cup chopped oil-packed sun-dried tomatoes

2 tablespoons pitted, sliced Kalamata olives

Juice of 1 lemon

2 tablespoons chopped fresh basil

1. Preheat the oven to 400°F. Line a baking sheet with parchment paper.

2. In a large bowl, toss together the squash, celery root, carrots, parsnips, and olive oil until coated. Season with salt and pepper.

3. Spread the vegetables on the baking sheet and roast until tender and lightly caramelized, turning once, about 40 minutes total.

4. Divide the roasted vegetables between bowls and top with the spinach, artichoke hearts, sun-dried tomatoes, and olives. Drizzle the bowls with lemon juice, top with basil, and serve.

PER SERVING: *Calories: 199; Total fat: 6g; Saturated fat: 1g; Carbohydrates: 37g; Sugar: 8g; Fiber: 8g; Protein: 4g*

Chicken with Yogurt-Mint Sauce

SERVES 4 • GLUTEN-FREE • MEAL IN ONE

PREP TIME:
10 MINUTES, PLUS
MARINATING TIME

COOK TIME:
25 MINUTES

Marinating chicken in yogurt is common in Greece and North Africa. Yogurt is the most effective tenderizer, better than vinegar or lemon-based marinades that can toughen protein. The calcium in the yogurt activates enzymes in the chicken that break down the protein. Thick Greek yogurt, rich in calcium, protein, and probiotics, is an excellent choice for this process.

1 cup low-fat plain Greek yogurt

¼ sweet onion, finely chopped

1 tablespoon chopped fresh mint

1 teaspoon chopped fresh dill

1 teaspoon minced garlic

1 teaspoon ground cumin

Pinch red pepper flakes

4 (3-ounce) boneless, skinless chicken breasts

1. In a medium bowl, whisk together the yogurt, onion, mint, dill, garlic, cumin, and red pepper flakes until blended. Transfer ½ cup of the yogurt to a small bowl. Set aside, covered, in the refrigerator.

2. Add the chicken to the remaining yogurt mixture, turning to coat. Cover and place the chicken in the refrigerator to marinate for 3 hours.

3. Preheat the oven to 400°F.

4. Transfer the chicken breasts to a baking sheet and roast until the chicken is cooked through, 20 to 25 minutes. Serve with the reserved yogurt-mint sauce.

PER SERVING: *Calories: 136; Total fat: 1g; Saturated fat: 0g; Carbohydrates: 5g; Sugar: 3g; Fiber: 1g; Protein: 26g*

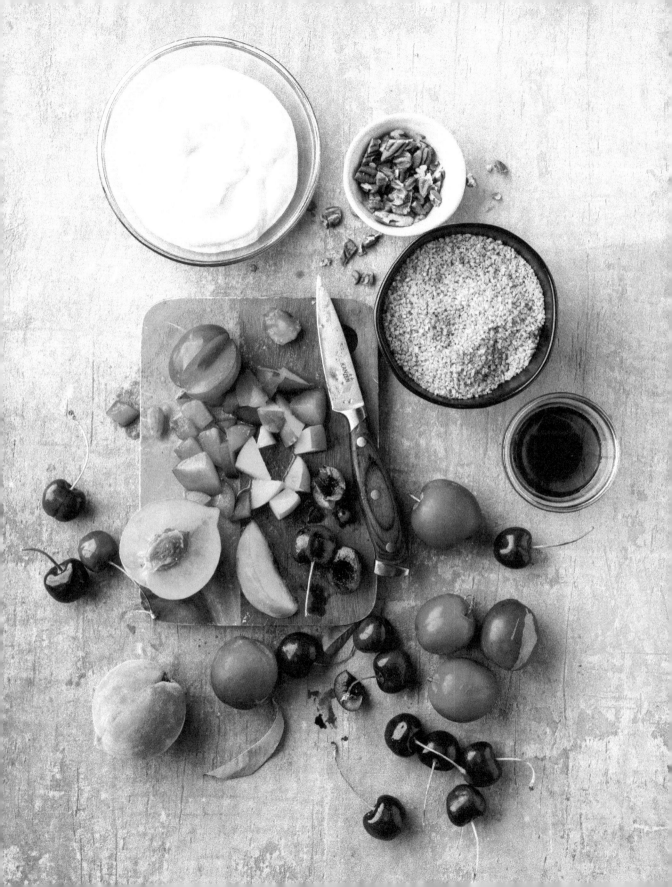

CHAPTER 5

Week Three Meal Plan and Recipes

Wow! You are at week three. Kudos to you for getting this far in the journey. Hopefully you are feeling more energized and are more focused at your work. You're probably wondering what's in store for you this week. Well, I am happy to report you are going to enjoy some delicious fruity breakfasts, a delectable shrimp and mint pesto pasta, and one of my favorites—tabbouleh. The Mediterranean diet is not just a diet; it really is a lifestyle change. So keep up the positive attitude, don't forget to get ample exercise as well as rest and relaxation, and nourish your body with the right foods this week.

WEEK THREE MEAL PLAN

	BREAKFAST	LUNCH	DINNER
MON	Fresh Fruit Crumble Muesli* (page 71)	*Leftover* Goat Cheese, Spinach, and Egg Frittata (from Week 2) with whole wheat pita	Whole-Wheat Spaghetti with Shrimp and Mint Pesto* (page 80)
TUE	*Leftover* Fresh Fruit Crumble Muesli	*Leftover* Whole-Wheat Spaghetti with Shrimp and Mint Pesto	Beet-Fennel Soup with Goat Cheese* (page 82)
WED	Stone Fruit Overnight Bulgur (page 72)	*Leftover* Beet-Fennel Soup with Goat Cheese	Sirloin with Sweet Bell Peppers* (page 83)
THU	Greek yogurt with strawberries and blueberries	*Leftover* Sirloin with Sweet Bell Peppers	Tabbouleh Pita Sandwich* (page 84)
FRI	Greek yogurt with peaches	*Leftover* Tabbouleh Pita Sandwich	Salmon Bowl with Bulgur and Tahini Sauce (page 85)
SAT	Egg White, Red Pepper, and Chard Scramble (page 73)	Greek Vegetable and Herb Pinwheels (page 77)	Halibut with Olive-Tomato Sauce (page 87)
SUN	Loaded Smoked Salmon Breakfast Casserole* (page 75)	Beet-Grapefruit Salad with Citrus-Basil Dressing (page 78)	Moroccan Spiced Chicken with Sweet Potato Hash (page 88)

These dishes will be eaten later as leftovers, so make extra if needed.

WEEK THREE SNACK IDEAS

GO NUTS: Mix your favorite nuts with dried fruit, including cranberries, dried apricots, raw almonds, walnuts, and raisins. Enjoy a ⅓-cup serving for a healthy and filling snack.

FETA CHEESE WITH WATERMELON BITES: Mix ¼ cup of diced watermelon and 1 ounce (about ¼ cup) of crumbled feta cheese. Enjoy by itself or with a plain brown rice cake.

WEEK THREE SHOPPING LIST

Canned and Bottled Items

- Almond milk, unsweetened (1½ cups)
- Coconut milk, light (1 [13.5-ounce] can)
- Pesto, sun-dried tomato or basil (¼ cup)
- Roasted red peppers (1 [6-ounce] jar)
- Salmon, canned, boneless, skinless (2 [5-ounce] cans)
- Stock, chicken, low-sodium (6 cups)

Dairy and Eggs

- Cheese, goat, crumbled (4 ounces)
- Cheese, Parmesan, grated (½ ounce)
- Cheese, ricotta (4 ounces)
- Eggs, large (22)
- Yogurt, plain, low-fat, Greek (4 cups)

Frozen

- Black cherries, pitted (1 cup)
- Edamame, shelled (1 cup)

Meat

- Beef, top sirloin steak, boneless (12 ounces)
- Chicken, breast, boneless, skinless (4 [3-ounce] pieces)
- Halibut (4 [4-ounce] fillets)
- Salmon, smoked (6 ounces)
- Shrimp (12 ounces)

Pantry Items

- Almonds
- Black pepper, ground
- Bulgur
- Bulgur, instant
- Cinnamon, ground
- Coriander, ground
- Cumin, ground
- Dates, Medjool
- Garlic powder
- Ginger, ground
- Maple syrup
- Nutmeg, ground
- Oats, rolled, gluten-free
- Oil, olive
- Pecans, halved
- Pine nuts
- Quinoa
- Red pepper flakes
- Sea salt
- Spaghetti, whole-wheat
- Tahini
- Vanilla extract
- Vinegar, apple cider

Produce

- Basil (1 large bunch)
- Beets (12)
- Bell pepper, orange (1)
- Bell peppers, red (5)
- Bell peppers, yellow (3)
- Blueberries (½ cup)
- Broccoli (2 small heads)
- Carrot (1)
- Cucumbers, English (2)
- Dill (1 bunch)
- Fennel (1 bulb)
- Garlic (1 head)
- Grapefruits, ruby red (2)
- Green beans (10 ounces)

- Kale, spinach, beet greens, or Swiss chard (12 ounces)
- Kale (4 ounces)
- Kiwis (2)
- Lemons (3)
- Lettuce, romaine (2 heads)
- Limes (2)
- Mint (1 bunch)
- Nectarine (1)
- Onions, red (2)
- Onions, sweet (3)
- Orange (1)
- Oregano (1 bunch)
- Parsley (2 bunches)
- Peach (1)
- Plums (3)
- Radishes (1 bunch)
- Scallions (1 bunch)
- Spinach (2 ounces)
- Strawberries (1 cup)
- Sweet potatoes (1 pound)
- Swiss chard (1 bunch)
- Tomatoes (4)
- Tomatoes, cherry (1 cup)
- Tomatoes, plum (2)
- Zucchini, green (1)
- Zucchini, yellow (1)

Other

- Olives, Kalamata, pitted (¼ cup)
- Pita bread rounds, whole-wheat (4)
- Tortillas, whole-grain (4)

WEEK THREE OPTIONAL PREP GUIDE

Wash and Cut

- Broccoli: chop
- Carrot: thinly slice
- Fennel: coarsely chop

- Kale, spinach, beet greens, or Swiss chard: chop
- Orange bell pepper: cut into thin strips
- Radishes: quarter
- Red bell pepper: chop 3, cut 2 into thin strips
- Romaine lettuce: shred
- Spinach: shred
- Swiss chard: shred
- Yellow bell pepper: chop 1, cut 2 into thin strips
- Yellow zucchini: halve lengthwise and thinly slice
- Zucchini: chop

Cook and Store

- Bulgur: 1 cup

Make Ahead

- Stone Fruit Overnight Bulgur (page 72)
- Mint Pesto (page 80)
- Tzatziki Sauce (page 192)

WEEK THREE RECIPE LIST

- Fresh Fruit Crumble Muesli
- Stone Fruit Overnight Bulgur
- Egg White, Red Pepper, and Chard Scramble
- Loaded Smoked Salmon Breakfast Casserole
- Greek Vegetable and Herb Pinwheels
- Beet-Grapefruit Salad with Citrus-Basil Dressing
- Whole-Wheat Spaghetti with Shrimp and Mint Pesto
- Beet-Fennel Soup with Goat Cheese
- Sirloin with Sweet Bell Peppers
- Tabbouleh Pita Sandwich
- Salmon Bowl with Bulgur and Tahini Sauce
- Halibut with Olive-Tomato Sauce
- Moroccan Spiced Chicken with Sweet Potato Hash

Fresh Fruit Crumble Muesli

SERVES 4 • GLUTEN-FREE • MEAL IN ONE • VEGETARIAN • 30 MINUTES OR LESS

PREP TIME:
20 MINUTES

You might think you are eating dessert for breakfast when you take your first luscious bite of the sweet fruit and rich, nutty topping in this recipe. You can change the mixture of fruit to anything you happen to have on hand. The pecans in the topping can help reduce inflammation in the body, support a healthy cardiovascular system, and improve brain function.

1 cup gluten-free rolled oats

¼ cup chopped pecans

¼ cup almonds

4 pitted Medjool dates

1 teaspoon vanilla extract

¼ teaspoon ground cinnamon

1 cup sliced fresh strawberries

1 nectarine, pitted and chopped

2 kiwis, peeled and chopped

½ cup blueberries

1 cup low-fat plain Greek yogurt

1. In a food processor, combine the oats, pecans, almonds, dates, vanilla, and cinnamon and pulse until the mixture resembles coarse crumbs.

2. In a medium bowl, stir together the strawberries, nectarine, kiwis, and blueberries until well mixed. Divide the fruit and yogurt between bowls and top each bowl with the oat mixture. Serve.

SUBSTITUTION TIP: *Many grocery stores carry date paste in the baking section, which is less expensive than whole dates. If you are puréeing or blending the fruit with other ingredients, as in this recipe, the date paste is a great alternative.*

PER SERVING: *Calories: 258; Total fat: 6g; Saturated fat: 0g; Carbohydrates: 45g; Sugar: 28g; Fiber: 7g; Protein: 11g*

Stone Fruit Overnight Bulgur

SERVES 4 • MEAL IN ONE • VEGETARIAN

PREP TIME:
15 MINUTES,
PLUS 8 HOURS
CHILLING TIME

Plums are the centerpiece of this hearty, flavor-packed meal. Plums are found in Turkey, Greece, Italy, and the south of France in all varieties and colors including green, yellow, purple, black, and red. If you want extra sweetness, choose yellow or black plums. This plump stone fruit is rich in pectin, fiber, calcium, potassium, and vitamins A, B, C, and K, which help it improve iron absorption and cut the risk of macular degeneration, high blood pressure, and cataracts. Make sure you leave the skin on the plums because it's packed with antioxidants.

2 cups low-fat plain Greek yogurt

1 cup instant bulgur

½ cup light coconut milk

¼ cup chopped pecans

¼ cup maple syrup

½ teaspoon ground ginger

3 plums, pitted and chopped

1 peach, pitted and chopped

1 cup pitted frozen or fresh black cherries

1. In a large bowl, stir together the yogurt, bulgur, coconut milk, pecans, maple syrup, and ginger until well mixed.

2. Evenly divide the mixture between bowls and top with the plums, peaches, and cherries. Cover the bowls and refrigerate overnight. Serve.

SUBSTITUTION TIP: *For a gluten-free version, you can replace bulgur with oats or steel-cut oats in the same amount. Make sure your oats have a label on the package stipulating that they are not manufactured in a plant with other gluten-containing grains.*

PER SERVING: *Calories: 321; Total fat: 4g; Saturated fat: 2g; Carbohydrates: 59g; Sugar: 27g; Fiber: 8g; Protein: 18g*

Egg White, Red Pepper, and Chard Scramble

SERVES 4 • DAIRY-FREE • GLUTEN-FREE • MEAL IN ONE • VEGETARIAN • 30 MINUTES OR LESS

PREP TIME:
10 MINUTES

COOK TIME:
15 MINUTES

Snowy white fluffy egg whites, deep green chard, and bright bell peppers combine for an ideal breakfast that can be eaten alone, with some fresh fruit, or stuffed into a whole-grain tortilla or pita. Egg white is very high in protein, low in fat, and contains no cholesterol, making it a perfect choice if you are watching calories. You can throw a few whole eggs into this scramble (try 8 whites and 4 whole eggs) to gain important nutrients like choline, which can help boost the metabolism.

12 large egg whites

½ cup unsweetened almond milk

¼ teaspoon ground nutmeg

Sea salt

Freshly ground black pepper

1 tablespoon olive oil

1 red bell pepper, chopped

½ sweet onion, chopped

1 teaspoon minced garlic

2 cups shredded Swiss chard

1 tablespoon chopped fresh parsley

1. In a medium bowl, whisk the egg whites, almond milk, and nutmeg until combined. Season lightly with salt and pepper and set aside.

2. In a large skillet, heat the olive oil over medium-high heat and sauté the bell pepper, onion, and garlic until softened, about 4 minutes. Stir in the chard and sauté until wilted, about 3 minutes more.

Continued >

Egg White, Red Pepper, and Chard Scramble

Continued

3. Reduce the heat to medium and pour the egg white mixture into the skillet. Scramble the egg whites with the vegetables, creating fluffy thick curds, until the egg whites are moist but cooked through, about 4 minutes. Serve topped with parsley.

INGREDIENT TIP: *Nutmeg has a warm, almost sweet taste that can be slightly lost in pre-ground jarred products. Whenever possible, purchase whole nutmeg kernels and grate your own. If you love nutmeg in your recipes, invest in a mill or microplane specifically designed for this spice.*

PER SERVING: *Calories: 107; Total fat: 4g; Saturated fat: 1g; Carbohydrates: 6g; Sugar: 3g; Fiber: 1g; Protein: 12g*

Loaded Smoked Salmon Breakfast Casserole

SERVES 6 • DAIRY-FREE • GLUTEN-FREE • MEAL IN ONE

PREP TIME:
10 MINUTES

COOK TIME:
45 MINUTES

Eggs and smoked salmon are an inspired flavor and nutritional pairing. These creamy dill-accented eggs seem infused with the luscious smoky flavor of the salmon in this easy-to-prepare casserole. Eggs contain nine amino acids and the antioxidants lutein and zeaxanthin, so they are extremely good for the eyes and can help prevent cataracts. Smoked salmon is good for the eyes as well, containing macular degeneration–preventing omega-3 fatty acids, heart-friendly protein, and B and D vitamins.

2 tablespoons olive oil

2 cups chopped fresh broccoli

1 sweet onion, chopped

1 red bell pepper, chopped

2 teaspoons minced garlic

10 large eggs, beaten

1 cup unsweetened almond milk

1 tablespoon chopped fresh dill

Sea salt

Freshly ground black pepper

6 ounces smoked salmon, chopped

1. Preheat the oven to 350°F.

2. In a large skillet, heat the olive oil over medium-high heat. Sauté the broccoli, onion, bell pepper, and garlic until softened, about 5 minutes.

3. Meanwhile, in a medium bowl, whisk together the eggs, almond milk, and dill until well blended and season with salt and pepper.

Continued >

Loaded Smoked Salmon Breakfast Casserole

Continued

4. Transfer the vegetable mixture to a 9-by-13-inch baking dish and top with the smoked salmon. Pour the egg mixture over the salmon and vegetables.

5. Bake, uncovered, until a knife inserted in the center comes out clean and the casserole is golden, 35 to 40 minutes. Serve.

INGREDIENT TIP: *Look for broccoli that has tight buds with no flowering or yellowing and a dry, crack-free stalk. Store broccoli in a sealed bag with all the air squeezed out in the refrigerator for up to 10 days.*

PER SERVING: *Calories: 226; Total fat: 15g; Saturated fat: 4g; Carbohydrates: 7g; Sugar: 3g; Fiber: 2g; Protein: 17g*

Greek Vegetable and Herb Pinwheels

SERVES 4 • MEAL IN ONE • VEGETARIAN • 30 MINUTES OR LESS

PREP TIME:
25 MINUTES

The term "pinwheel" conjures up festive images of colorful toys and spirals, which is what this pretty wrap will remind you of. Carrots are a vibrant addition to the mixture, bright and crisp. You can look for different-color carrots for visual impact, such as orange, red, purple, white, and yellow. Each color contains different antioxidants like beta-carotene (orange), xanthophyll (yellow), lycopene (red), and anthocyanin (purple). These powerful antioxidants promote eye and immune system health and help fight heart disease and cancer.

4 whole-grain tortillas

¼ cup store-bought sun-dried tomato pesto or basil pesto

½ cup ricotta cheese

1 cup shredded spinach

1 red bell pepper, thinly sliced

1 yellow bell pepper, thinly sliced

1 carrot, thinly sliced

¼ cup chopped basil

1. On each tortilla, spread about 1 tablespoon of pesto up to about 1 inch from the edge.

2. Evenly divide the ricotta between the tortillas and spread it out in the center. Divide the spinach, bell peppers, carrot, and basil between the tortillas. Tightly roll the tortillas and cut into pinwheels. Serve.

SUBSTITUTION TIP: *Ricotta cheese adds a lovely tanginess to this wrap but can be replaced with a non-dairy option or hummus if you want a vegan lunch. Or you can leave it out completely and add more vegetables or a handful of legumes for extra flavor.*

PER SERVING: *Calories: 274; Total fat: 14g; Saturated fat: 4g; Carbohydrates: 30g; Sugar: 2g; Fiber: 3g; Protein: 13g*

Beet-Grapefruit Salad with Citrus-Basil Dressing

SERVES 4 • GLUTEN-FREE • MEAL IN ONE • VEGETARIAN

PREP TIME:
20 MINUTES,
PLUS 2 HOURS
CHILLING TIME

——————

COOK TIME:
20 MINUTES

——————

You might consider this one of the loveliest salads you have ever eaten with its deep reds, pink, dark green, and soft white. Ruby red grapefruit has the highest number of antioxidants of all grapefruits due to its deep color. It also contains vitamins A and C, D-glucaric acid, calcium, pectin, potassium, thiamine, folate, and phosphorus. Grapefruit can cleanse the lymphatic system, stimulate digestion, and reduce the risk of osteoporosis and cancer.

FOR THE DRESSING

¼ cup olive oil

2 tablespoons freshly squeezed orange juice

1 tablespoon apple cider vinegar

Juice and zest of 1 lime

1 tablespoon chopped fresh basil

Sea salt

Freshly ground black pepper

FOR THE SALAD

6 beets, peeled and cut in half

1 teaspoon olive oil

6 cups chopped mixed greens (kale, spinach, beet greens, or Swiss chard)

2 large ruby red grapefruits, peeled, pith removed, segmented, and cut into chunks

1 scallion, both white and green parts, sliced

½ cup chopped pecans

½ cup crumbled goat cheese

In a small bowl, whisk together the olive oil, orange juice, vinegar, lime juice, lime zest, and basil. Season with salt and pepper and set aside.

TO MAKE THE SALAD

1. Preheat the oven to 400°F.

2. In an 8-by-8-inch baking dish, toss the beets with the olive oil. Roast until the beets are tender, about 20 minutes.

3. Remove the beets from the oven and chill them in the refrigerator, about 2 hours. Cut the beets into wedges.

4. In a large bowl, toss the greens together with half of the dressing until well coated. Evenly divide the greens between serving plates. Top each salad with beet wedges, grapefruits, scallion, pecans, and goat cheese.

5. Evenly drizzle the remaining dressing over the salads and serve.

SUBSTITUTION TIP: *For an interesting variation on basil, try tarragon. This lovely herb has a licorice flavor and should only be used fresh. Unfortunately, dried tarragon loses its essential oils, which means less flavor. Any leftover tarragon can be used in other recipes or frozen and stored in sealed plastic bags for up to 1 month.*

PER SERVING: *Calories: 355; Total fat: 24g; Saturated fat: 6g; Carbohydrates: 32g; Sugar: 25g; Fiber: 6g; Protein: 9g*

Whole-Wheat Spaghetti with Shrimp and Mint Pesto

SERVES 4 • MEAL IN ONE

PREP TIME:
10 MINUTES

COOK TIME:
30 MINUTES

Mint and lime add a pleasing freshness to pesto, which is especially lovely with sweet shrimp. Mint's distinctive cool flavor comes from a component called menthol, which can help calm gastrointestinal issues and reduce inflammation in the body. Mint is a great source of vitamins A, B$_2$, and C, iron, calcium, copper, and potassium. Mint can promote liver health, cleanse the blood, fight the common cold, and reduce the risk of cancer.

FOR THE PESTO

½ cup fresh mint leaves

½ cup fresh basil leaves

¼ cup pine nuts

2 tablespoons grated Parmesan cheese

1 tablespoon freshly squeezed lime juice

1 tablespoon olive oil

FOR THE PASTA

8 ounces whole-wheat spaghetti

1 tablespoon olive oil

12 ounces cooked, peeled shrimp

1 yellow zucchini, cut lengthwise and thinly sliced

2 cups green beans, cut into 1-inch pieces

Sea salt

TO MAKE THE PESTO

In a food processor, combine the mint, basil, pine nuts, Parmesan cheese, lime juice, and olive oil and pulse until a chunky paste forms. Transfer to a bowl and set aside.

TO MAKE THE PASTA

1. Bring a large pot of water to a boil and cook the pasta according to package directions until al dente. Drain.

2. In a large skillet, heat the olive oil over medium-high heat. Sauté the shrimp until heated through, stirring occasionally, 5 to 7 minutes.

3. Add the zucchini and green beans to the skillet and sauté for 3 to 4 minutes more. Remove from the heat and add the cooked pasta and the pesto to the skillet, tossing to combine. Season with salt and serve.

INGREDIENT TIP: *This recipe calls for cooked shrimp, so you can easily utilize frozen products to save a bit of money with no loss of quality. Thaw the shrimp overnight in the refrigerator and use whatever size suits you for this dish, large (31 to 35 count) or small (51 to 60 count), and adjust the cooking time in step 2 depending on your choice.*

PER SERVING: *Calories: 453; Total fat: 16g; Saturated fat: 3g; Carbohydrates: 50g; Sugar: 2g; Fiber: 2g; Protein: 32g*

Beet-Fennel Soup with Goat Cheese

SERVES 4 • GLUTEN-FREE • MEAL IN ONE

PREP TIME:
10 MINUTES

COOK TIME:
30 MINUTES

Beets and fennel are a classic combination—the earthy sweetness of the beets and licorice-flavored fennel make for a sublime pairing. Beets are an extraordinary color, especially if you use deep ruby red or stunning vibrant yellow varieties. Expect many health benefits from consuming beets, such as reducing the impact of anemia by rebuilding blood cells, lowering blood pressure, detoxifying the liver, and promoting gallbladder health.

1 tablespoon olive oil

6 large beets, peeled and chopped

1 fennel bulb, coarsely chopped

1 sweet onion, chopped

1 teaspoon minced garlic

6 cups low-sodium chicken stock

Sea salt

Freshly ground black pepper

½ cup crumbled goat cheese

1 tablespoon chopped fresh parsley

1. In a large pot, heat the olive oil over medium-high heat. Sauté the beets, fennel, onion, and garlic until they soften, stirring occasionally, about 10 minutes.

2. Add the chicken stock and bring the soup to a boil. Reduce the heat to low and simmer until the vegetables are very tender, about 20 minutes.

3. Transfer the soup to a food processor or, using an immersion blender, purée until smooth. Return the soup to the saucepan and season with salt and pepper. Serve topped with goat cheese and parsley.

PER SERVING: *Calories: 309; Total fat: 13g; Saturated fat: 5g; Carbohydrates: 32g; Sugar: 17g; Fiber: 5g; Protein: 17g*

Sirloin with Sweet Bell Peppers

SERVES 4 • DAIRY-FREE • GLUTEN-FREE • 30 MINUTES OR LESS

PREP TIME:
20 MINUTES

COOK TIME:
8 MINUTES

This sheet-pan recipe creates Greek-inspired fajitas. Double the recipe and wrap the meat and veggies in a whole-grain tortilla for a quick lunch the next day. Sirloin steak is lower in fat than many other cuts of beef, making it a good choice for the Mediterranean diet.

12 ounces boneless top sirloin steak, about 1-inch thick, trimmed of visible fat

1 tablespoon olive oil, divided

Sea salt

Freshly ground black pepper

1 yellow bell pepper, thinly sliced

1 red bell pepper, thinly sliced

1 orange bell pepper, thinly sliced

1 small red onion, thinly sliced

4 garlic cloves, crushed

Juice of 1 lemon

1. Preheat the oven to broil.

2. Lightly oil the steak on both sides with 1 teaspoon of olive oil and season with salt and pepper. Place the steak on a baking sheet.

3. In a large bowl, toss together the bell peppers, onion, garlic, and remaining 2 teaspoons of olive oil. Season lightly with salt and pepper. Spread the vegetables on the baking sheet around the steak.

4. Broil the steak and vegetables until the steak is browned and the desired doneness, turning once, about 4 minutes per side.

5. Remove from the oven and let the steak rest for 10 minutes. Slice thinly on the bias against the grain. Drizzle the vegetables with lemon juice and serve.

PER SERVING: *Calories: 170; Total fat: 7g; Saturated fat: 2g; Carbohydrates: 11g; Sugar: 2g; Fiber: 2g; Protein: 18g*

Tabbouleh Pita Sandwich

SERVES 4 • MEAL IN ONE • VEGETARIAN

PREP TIME:
20 MINUTES, PLUS
COOLING TIME

COOK TIME:
15 MINUTES

Pitas are a nutritious container for almost any filling. Whole-grain pita bread has fewer carbs than many other bread choices, and is relatively low in fat and high in protein. The filling will add heaps of healthy fiber, vitamins, and minerals for a satisfying, nutritious lunch.

1 cup quinoa

2 cups water

½ English cucumber, chopped

1 cup halved cherry tomatoes

1 yellow bell pepper, chopped

1 scallion, both white and green parts, chopped

½ cup chopped fresh parsley

Juice and zest of 1 lemon

2 tablespoons olive oil

1 teaspoon minced garlic

Sea salt

4 whole-wheat pitas

½ cup Tzatziki Sauce (page 192)

1. Rinse the quinoa under cold running water to remove its bitter flavor. In a small saucepan, combine the quinoa and water and bring to a boil over medium heat. Reduce the heat to low and simmer, uncovered, until the liquid is absorbed, 10 to 15 minutes. Transfer to a dish and refrigerate until cool.

2. In a large bowl, stir together the cooled quinoa, cucumber, tomatoes, bell pepper, scallion, parsley, lemon juice, lemon zest, olive oil, and garlic until well mixed. Season with salt.

3. Cut the pitas in half and split them open. Spoon the quinoa mixture evenly into the pita halves. Top with tzatziki sauce and serve.

PER SERVING: *Calories: 288; Total fat: 10g; Saturated fat: 1g; Carbohydrates: 43g; Sugar: 5g; Fiber: 6g; Protein: 10g*

Salmon Bowl with Bulgur and Tahini Sauce

SERVES 4 • DAIRY-FREE • MEAL IN ONE

PREP TIME:
20 MINUTES, PLUS
2 HOURS
CHILLING TIME

COOK TIME:
15 MINUTES

If you are looking for a little heat in your meal or a different flavor from the commonly used Mediterranean vegetables, pick up a zesty bunch of radishes. Depending on your choice, the heat in a radish ranges from searing hot to mild and peppery. Radishes contain phosphorus, potassium, copper, zinc, and vitamins A, B, and C, so they are great detoxifiers and can help relieve digestive issues and reduce the risk of kidney stones.

FOR THE TAHINI SAUCE

¼ cup light coconut milk

¼ cup tahini

2 tablespoons freshly squeezed lemon juice

¼ teaspoon garlic powder

¼ teaspoon ground cumin

Sea salt

FOR THE SALMON BOWL

1 cup bulgur

2 cups water

4 cups shredded romaine lettuce

2 (5-ounce) cans boneless, skinless salmon, drained

1 cup shelled frozen edamame, thawed

2 plum tomatoes, sliced

10 radishes, quartered

2 scallions, both white and green parts, thinly sliced

TO MAKE THE TAHINI SAUCE

In a small bowl, whisk together the coconut milk, tahini, lemon juice, garlic powder, and cumin until blended. Season with salt and set aside.

Continued >

Salmon Bowl with Bulgur and Tahini Sauce

Continued

TO MAKE THE SALMON BOWL

1. In a pot, combine the bulgur and water. Bring to a boil, cover, and reduce the heat to simmer for 12 to 15 minutes, until tender. Drain any excess liquid, transfer to a bowl, and chill in the refrigerator for 2 hours.

2. Divide the romaine between bowls and top each with bulgur, salmon, edamame, tomatoes, radishes, and scallions. Drizzle with tahini sauce and serve.

INGREDIENT TIP: *If you want to boost the nutritional impact of this dish, try adding radish leaves along with the shredded romaine. Radish leaves are packed with protein and vitamins, even more than the radish root, which is an excellent source of vitamin C and fiber.*

PER SERVING: *Calories: 378; Total fat: 16g; Saturated fat: 3g; Carbohydrates: 38g; Sugar: 4g; Fiber: 10g; Protein: 26g*

Halibut with Olive-Tomato Sauce

SERVES 4 • DAIRY-FREE • GLUTEN-FREE

PREP TIME:
15 MINUTES

COOK TIME:
25 MINUTES

Cumin provides a peppery, citrusy, and nutty flavor to this recipe's sauce. Cumin is high in iron and is a good source of magnesium, calcium, and manganese.

4 (4-ounce) halibut fillets

2 teaspoons ground cumin

Sea salt

1 tablespoon olive oil, divided

½ red onion, thinly sliced

2 teaspoons minced garlic

4 large tomatoes, chopped

½ cup chopped roasted red peppers

¼ cup pitted, chopped Kalamata olives

1 tablespoon chopped fresh oregano

Pinch red pepper flakes

1 tablespoon chopped fresh parsley

1. Season the halibut with cumin and salt.

2. In a large skillet, heat 2 teaspoons of olive oil over medium-high heat. Cook the fish until it flakes easily, turning once, about 12 minutes total. Set aside.

3. Add the remaining 1 teaspoon of olive oil to the skillet and sauté the onion and garlic until softened, about 2 minutes.

4. Stir in the tomatoes, roasted red peppers, olives, oregano, and red pepper flakes and reduce the heat to medium low. Cook, stirring, until the sauce is well blended and heated through, about 10 minutes. Serve the fish topped with sauce and parsley.

PER SERVING: *Calories: 219; Total fat: 8g; Saturated fat: 1g; Carbohydrates: 12g; Sugar: 7g; Fiber: 4g; Protein: 28g*

Moroccan Spiced Chicken with Sweet Potato Hash

SERVES 4 • DAIRY-FREE • GLUTEN-FREE • MEAL IN ONE

PREP TIME:
15 MINUTES

COOK TIME:
40 MINUTES

Sweet potatoes are one of those ingredients that seem to perk up with the addition of spices, especially the warm ones associated with North African cooking. The sweetness and depth of the tuber create a sublime balance with the chicken and earthy kale in this dish. Sweet potatoes add vitamins A, C, and E, beta-carotene, calcium, iron, potassium, and folic acid to your diet. This means stabilized blood sugar, a reduction in the risk of cancer, and a healthy digestive system.

¼ teaspoon ground cumin

¼ teaspoon ground coriander

¼ teaspoon ground ginger

¼ teaspoon ground cinnamon

4 (3-ounce) boneless, skinless chicken breasts

2 tablespoons olive oil, divided

1 pound sweet potatoes, peeled and cut into ½-inch cubes

1 red bell pepper, chopped

1 zucchini, chopped

½ sweet onion, chopped

2 teaspoons minced garlic

2 cups stemmed, chopped kale

Sea salt

Freshly ground black pepper

1. In a small bowl, stir together the cumin, coriander, ginger, and cinnamon. Dredge the chicken breasts in the spices so they are well coated.

2. In a large skillet, heat 1 tablespoon of olive oil over medium-high heat. Pan-fry the chicken until completely cooked through, turning once, about 15 minutes total.

3. Transfer the chicken to a plate and cover with aluminum foil to keep warm.

4. Add the remaining 1 tablespoon of olive oil to the skillet and sauté the sweet potatoes until tender, about 15 minutes.

5. Add the bell pepper, zucchini, onion, and garlic and sauté until the vegetables are softened and heated through, stirring occasionally, about 5 minutes.

6. Add the kale and sauté until wilted, about 4 minutes more. Season with salt and pepper. Evenly divide between plates, top each with a chicken breast, and serve.

SUBSTITUTION TIP: *Sweet potatoes are not a traditional ingredient in Moroccan cuisine, but they taste delicious and are readily available in any store. Try using diced pumpkin instead, fresh or frozen, in the same amount, to create a true North African dish.*

PER SERVING: *Calories: 277; Total fat: 8g; Saturated fat: 1g; Carbohydrates: 29g; Sugar: 7g; Fiber: 5g; Protein: 23g*

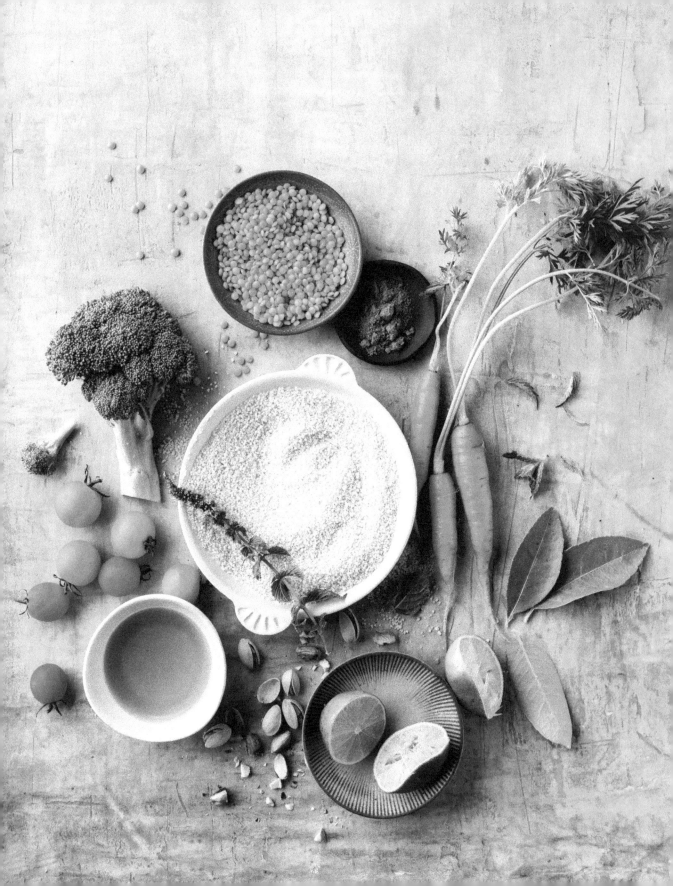

CHAPTER 6

Week Four
Meal Plan and Recipes

Look at you! You're in your final week of the four-week plan. You must be feeling quite proud right now; you are feeling energized and looking good. You've become an expert at what you can eat on the Mediterranean diet, and have likely realized that this is a sustainable diet you can follow for life without feeling like you're constantly restricting your calories or denying yourself delicious foods. This week the vibrancy and variety of the Mediterranean palate will come to life with Greek-Style Tuna Salad in Pita (page 100), Chicken Shawarma Bowls (page 112), and Barley Risotto with Sweet Potato and Spinach (page 110).

WEEK FOUR MEAL PLAN

	BREAKFAST	LUNCH	DINNER
MON	*Leftover* Loaded Smoked Salmon Breakfast Casserole (from Week 3)	Greek-Style Tuna Salad in Pita* (page 100)	Hummus-Crusted Halibut (page 103) Moroccan Couscous Salad* (page 104)
TUE	Overnight Steel-Cut Oats Porridge with Cherries* (page 95)	*Leftover* Greek-Style Tuna Salad in Pita	North African Chicken Apricot Tagine* (page 106)
WED	*Leftover* Overnight Steel-Cut Oats Porridge with Cherries	*Leftover* Moroccan Couscous Salad	Baking Sheet Spicy Shrimp with Vegetables (page 108)
THU	Avocado-Blueberry Smoothie (page 96)	*Leftover* North African Chicken Apricot Tagine	Chickpea Veggie Burgers* (page 109) served with pita
FRI	Greek yogurt and berries	*Leftover* Chickpea Veggie Burgers, served with pita	Barley Risotto with Sweet Potato and Spinach* (page 110)
SAT	California Egg White Scramble (page 97)	*Leftover* Barley Risotto with Sweet Potato and Spinach	Tunisian Herb Chicken Skewers (page 111)
SUN	Sun-dried Tomato and Asparagus Frittata (page 98)	Lemon-Spinach Salad with Pears and Blue Cheese (page 101)	Chicken Shawarma Bowls (page 112)

These dishes will be eaten later as leftovers, so make extra if needed.

WEEK FOUR SNACK IDEAS

CRANBERRY–PUMPKIN SEED TRAIL MIX:
This fiber-rich snack will help you stay full on
the go. Just throw about 2 tablespoons of dried
cranberries, 1 tablespoon of pumpkin seeds, and
1 tablespoon of raw almonds in a small reseal-
able bag.

TOMATO WITH MOZZARELLA CHEESE: Slice a
fresh tomato, drizzle lightly with olive oil, and top
with a slice of fresh mozzarella and a few sprigs
of basil.

WEEK FOUR SHOPPING LIST

Canned and Bottled Items

- Almond milk, vanilla, unsweetened (2½ cups)
- Chickpeas, low-sodium (4 [15.5-ounce] cans)
- Lentils, low-sodium (1 [15.5-ounce] can)
- Stock, vegetable, low-sodium (3 cups)
- Tomatoes, diced, low-sodium
  (1 [15-ounce] can)
- Tomatoes, sun-dried, oil-packed (¾ cup)
- Tuna, water-packed (2 [5-ounce] cans)

Dairy and Eggs

- Butter (1 tablespoon)
- Cheese, blue, crumbled (2 ounces)
- Cheese, feta, crumbled (2 ounces)
- Cheese, mozzarella, shredded (2 ounces)
- Cheese, Parmesan, grated (2 ounces)
- Eggs, large (21)
- Milk, low-fat (½ cup)
- Yogurt, plain, low-fat, Greek (1½ cups)

Frozen

- Black cherries, pitted (2 cups)

Meat

- Chicken, breast, boneless, skinless (3 pounds)
- Halibut (4 [4-ounce] fillets)
- Shrimp (1 pound)

Pantry Items

- Almonds, sliced
- Apricots, dried
- Barley, pearl
- Black pepper, ground
- Cardamom, ground
- Cayenne pepper, ground
- Chia seeds
- Chili powder
- Cinnamon, ground
- Coriander, ground
- Couscous
- Cranberries
- Cumin, ground
- Garlic powder
- Ginger, ground
- Honey
- Oats, rolled
- Oats, steel-cut
- Oil, olive
- Panko breadcrumbs, whole-wheat
- Paprika
- Paprika, smoked
- Pistachios, shelled
- Quinoa
- Sea salt
- Sunflower seeds
- Tahini
- Turmeric, ground
- Vanilla extract
- Walnuts

Produce

- Asparagus (2 bunches)
- Avocados (2)
- Baby bok choy (3)
- Basil (1 bunch)
- Bell pepper, red (1)
- Bell pepper, yellow (1)

- Blueberries (1 cup)
- Broccoli (2 small heads)
- Carrots (5)
- Cauliflower (1 small head)
- Celery (1 stalk)
- Cilantro (1 bunch)
- Cucumbers, English (2)
- Dill (1 bunch)
- Garlic (1 head)
- Ginger (1 small piece)
- Jalapeño (1)
- Lemons (7)
- Lettuce, Boston (1 head)
- Limes (3)
- Mint (1 bunch)
- Onion, red (1)
- Onions, sweet (3)
- Oregano (1 bunch)
- Parsley (1 bunch)
- Pears (2)
- Scallions (1 bunch)
- Spinach, baby (16 ounces)
- Sweet potatoes (2)
- Thyme (1 bunch)
- Tomatoes (2)
- Tomatoes, cherry (1 cup)
- Zucchini, yellow (1)

Other

- Olives, Kalamata, pitted (2 tablespoons)
- Pita bread rounds, whole-wheat (4)

WEEK FOUR OPTIONAL PREP GUIDE

Wash and Cut

- Asparagus: chop 2 cups, remove ends of remaining 10 spears and halve
- Boston lettuce: shred
- Broccoli: finely chop

- Carrot: peel and shred 3; cut lengthwise, then slice 2
- Cauliflower: cut into florets
- Celery: chop
- English cucumber: chop 1
- Red bell pepper: cut into thin strips
- Spinach: wash and dry all, shred 1 cup, store remaining leaves whole
- Yellow bell pepper: chop
- Zucchini, yellow: slice

Cook and Store

- Couscous: 1 cup
- Quinoa: 1 cup

Make Ahead

- Overnight Steel-Cut Oats Porridge with Cherries (page 95)
- Moroccan Couscous Salad (page 104)
- Tzatziki Sauce (page 192)

WEEK FOUR RECIPE LIST

- Overnight Steel-Cut Oats Porridge with Cherries
- Avocado-Blueberry Smoothie
- California Egg White Scramble
- Sun-dried Tomato and Asparagus Frittata
- Greek-Style Tuna Salad in Pita
- Lemon-Spinach Salad with Pears and Blue Cheese
- Hummus-Crusted Halibut
- Moroccan Couscous Salad
- North African Chicken Apricot Tagine
- Baking Sheet Spicy Shrimp with Vegetables
- Chickpea Veggie Burgers
- Barley Risotto with Sweet Potato and Spinach
- Tunisian Herb Chicken Skewers
- Chicken Shawarma Bowls

Overnight Steel-Cut Oats Porridge with Cherries

SERVES 4 • DAIRY-FREE • GLUTEN-FREE • MEAL IN ONE • VEGETARIAN

PREP TIME:
15 MINUTES,
PLUS 8 HOURS
CHILLING TIME

Cherries are cultivated in many Mediterranean countries. This luscious fruit can be pricey out of season, which runs from about May to September, but is worth every penny. Black cherries have the highest antioxidant levels and are associated with relieving arthritis pain and gout symptoms. They are an excellent source of folic acid and vitamins B, C, and E. Try including cherries in your diet to protect against urinary tract infections and cancer.

2 cups unsweetened vanilla almond milk

1 cup steel-cut oats

2 tablespoons chia seeds

2 tablespoons honey

¼ teaspoon ground cinnamon

2 cups frozen or fresh pitted black cherries

½ cup sliced almonds

¼ cup sunflower seeds

1. In a large bowl, stir together the almond milk, oats, chia seeds, honey, and cinnamon until well mixed. Cover the bowl and refrigerate overnight, stirring a few times.

2. Spoon the oats into bowls and top with cherries, almonds, and sunflower seeds. Serve.

SUBSTITUTION TIP: *Honey is not allowed on a strict vegan diet, so you can leave it out entirely or replace it with maple syrup. The cherries add natural sweetness, so you might find the dish to your taste without any sweetener at all.*

PER SERVING: *Calories: 296; Total fat: 13g; Saturated fat: 1g; Carbohydrates: 40g; Sugar: 17g; Fiber: 8g; Protein: 8g*

Avocado-Blueberry Smoothie

SERVES 2 • GLUTEN-FREE • MEAL IN ONE • VEGETARIAN • 30 MINUTES OR LESS

PREP TIME:
5 MINUTES

Some smoothies are snacks or a light breakfast, but you will be satisfied and full of energy with this combination of yogurt, avocado, oats, and sweet blueberries. Blueberries are ranked at the top of the list of produce for antioxidant capabilities. They are absolutely packed with phytonutrients, anti-inflammatories, calcium, iron, folic acid, and B vitamins. Enjoy blueberries several times a week to cut your risk of cancer, diabetes, bladder issues, heart disease, and cognitive diseases. Blueberries also help stabilize blood sugar and promote good eye health.

½ cup unsweetened vanilla almond milk

½ cup low-fat plain Greek yogurt

1 ripe avocado, peeled, pitted, and coarsely chopped

1 cup blueberries

¼ cup gluten-free rolled oats

½ teaspoon vanilla extract

4 ice cubes

1. In a blender, combine the almond milk, yogurt, avocado, blueberries, oats, and vanilla and pulse until well blended.

2. Add the ice cubes and blend until thick and smooth. Serve.

SUBSTITUTION TIP: *The yogurt can be omitted for those with dairy allergies or vegans. Try a couple tablespoons of coconut cream instead or a soy/ coconut yogurt for extra creaminess.*

PER SERVING: *Calories: 273; Total fat: 15g; Saturated fat: 2g; Carbohydrates: 28g; Sugar: 10g; Fiber: 9g; Protein: 10g*

California Egg White Scramble

SERVES 4 • DAIRY-FREE • GLUTEN-FREE • MEAL IN ONE • VEGETARIAN • 30 MINUTES OR LESS

PREP TIME:
20 MINUTES

COOK TIME:
5 MINUTES

Don't let this recipe's name fool you. Its ingredients—fresh herbs, olive oil, avocado, and tomatoes—are popular in the Mediterranean as well as in California for their high nutritional impact. Thyme supports a healthy digestive system, relieves respiratory conditions and arthritis, and detoxifies the liver.

10 large egg whites

1 tablespoon chopped fresh parsley

1 teaspoon chopped fresh basil

½ teaspoon chopped fresh thyme

Sea salt

Pinch freshly ground black pepper

1 tablespoon olive oil

1 ripe avocado, pitted, peeled, and chopped

1 cup halved cherry tomatoes, at room temperature

1 scallion, both white and green parts, thinly sliced on the bias

2 tablespoons chopped fresh cilantro

1 tablespoon minced jalapeño

1. In a medium bowl, whisk together the egg whites, parsley, basil, and thyme and season with salt and pepper.

2. In a large skillet, heat the olive oil over medium heat. Pour the egg mixture into the skillet and swirl the pan lightly. Scramble the eggs until cooked through but still moist, about 5 minutes.

3. Spoon the eggs onto a platter and top with avocado, tomatoes, scallion, cilantro, and jalapeño. Serve.

PER SERVING: *Calories: 156; Total fat: 10g; Saturated fat: 1g; Carbohydrates: 7g; Sugar: 2g; Fiber: 4g; Protein: 10g*

Sun-dried Tomato and Asparagus Frittata

SERVES 4 • GLUTEN-FREE • MEAL IN ONE • VEGETARIAN • 30 MINUTES OR LESS

PREP TIME:
10 MINUTES

COOK TIME:
20 MINUTES

Asparagus is a tender spring vegetable thought to have originated in eastern Mediterranean countries. In ancient Greece, asparagus was considered an aphrodisiac, so including it in a humble breakfast creation could be a good way to start your day. Asparagus has a strong flavor that is offset by sweet sun-dried tomato and creamy mozzarella. Asparagus packs a lot of nutrients in its slender stalks, including vitamins A, B, C, E, and K. It is also a source of protein, fiber, potassium, calcium, iron, and magnesium. Asparagus is great for detoxifying the body, improving kidney disorders, alleviating arthritis pain, and supporting cardiovascular health.

10 large eggs

½ cup low-fat milk

Sea salt

Dash freshly ground black pepper

1 tablespoon olive oil

2 cups chopped asparagus

½ cup chopped oil-packed sun-dried tomatoes

1 scallion, both white and green parts, chopped

½ cup shredded mozzarella

1 tablespoon chopped fresh basil

1. Preheat the oven to broil.

2. In a medium bowl, whisk together the eggs and milk and season with salt and pepper.

3. In a large ovenproof skillet, heat the olive oil over medium heat. Sauté the asparagus, sun-dried tomatoes, and scallion until softened, about 4 minutes.

4. Add the egg mixture to the skillet and cook until the edges are firm, and then lift the edges of the cooked egg to allow the uncooked egg to flow underneath until the eggs are nearly cooked through, about 10 minutes.

5. Remove from the heat and sprinkle the top with mozzarella. Place the skillet in the oven and broil until the cheese is melted and the frittata is cooked through, about 2 minutes. Cut into wedges and serve topped with basil.

COOKING TIP: *For a convenient meal, you can cut the frittata into wedges after it has cooled and store them in the freezer in sealed plastic bags for up to 1 month. Defrost the frittata in the refrigerator over-night when you wish to eat it.*

PER SERVING: *Calories: 304; Total fat: 20g; Saturated fat: 7g; Carbohydrates: 10g; Sugar: 6g; Fiber: 3g; Protein: 23g*

Greek-Style Tuna Salad in Pita

SERVES 4 • MEAL IN ONE • 30 MINUTES OR LESS

PREP TIME:
25 MINUTES

This is not the humble tuna sandwich you may have packed in school lunches. Instead, it is lemony and stuffed with rich olives, sun-dried tomatoes, and juicy cucumber chunks. You can use the more readily available mixed greens, romaine, or baby spinach instead of Boston lettuce. Black olives will work if you can't find Kalamata olives.

2 (5-ounce) cans water-packed tuna, drained

½ English cucumber, chopped

1 yellow bell pepper, chopped

¼ cup chopped oil-packed sun-dried tomatoes

2 tablespoons pitted, chopped Kalamata olives

2 tablespoons chopped fresh parsley

1 tablespoon freshly squeezed lemon juice

Sea salt

Freshly ground black pepper

4 whole-wheat pita bread rounds, halved

½ cup crumbled feta cheese

1 cup shredded Boston lettuce

1. In a large bowl, stir together the tuna, cucumber, bell pepper, sun-dried tomatoes, olives, parsley, and lemon juice. Season with salt and pepper.

2. Scoop the tuna salad into the pita halves and top them with feta cheese and lettuce. Serve.

PER SERVING: *Calories: 192; Total fat: 6g; Saturated fat: 3g; Carbohydrates: 23g; Sugar: 5g; Fiber: 3g; Protein: 14g*

Lemon-Spinach Salad with Pears and Blue Cheese

SERVES 4 • GLUTEN-FREE • MEAL IN ONE • VEGETARIAN • 30 MINUTES OR LESS

PREP TIME:
25 MINUTES

Pears and blue cheese are a classic French pairing found in appetizers, desserts, and salads like this citrus-brightened preparation. The sweetness of the pear is offset by the tangy sharpness of the cheese, creating magic. Pears are a fabulous source of vitamins B, C, and E, as well as pectin, potassium, and copper. This elegant fruit also contains a fruit sugar called levulose that people with diabetes can handle better than other sugars. Pears can help prevent and alleviate constipation, detoxify the body, lower cholesterol, and support neurological health.

FOR THE DRESSING

¼ cup olive oil

2 tablespoons freshly squeezed lemon juice

Zest of ¼ lemon

2 teaspoons honey

½ teaspoon chopped fresh thyme

Sea salt

Pinch freshly ground black pepper

FOR THE SALAD

6 cups baby spinach

¼ red onion, very thinly sliced

2 pears, cored and chopped

½ cup crumbled blue cheese

¼ cup dried cranberries

2 tablespoons chopped walnuts

TO MAKE THE DRESSING

In a small bowl, whisk together the olive oil, lemon juice, lemon zest, honey, and thyme. Season with salt and pepper and set aside.

Continued >

Lemon-Spinach Salad with Pears and Blue Cheese

Continued

TO MAKE THE SALAD

1. In a large bowl, toss together the spinach and dressing.

2. Evenly divide the spinach between plates and top each with onion, pears, blue cheese, cranberries, and walnuts. Serve.

INGREDIENT TIP: *Blue cheese can be an acquired taste; if you like a milder blue cheese, try Danish blue or Gorgonzola, and if your palate leans toward stronger flavor, top this salad with Stilton or Roquefort.*

PER SERVING: *Calories: 267; Total fat: 18g; Saturated fat: 5g; Carbohydrates: 25g; Sugar: 17g; Fiber: 5g; Protein: 5g*

Hummus-Crusted Halibut

SERVES 4 • DAIRY-FREE • 30 MINUTES OR LESS

PREP TIME:
10 MINUTES

COOK TIME:
15 MINUTES

Hummus and fresh, flaky fish make a tender, garlicky main course. The hummus crumb topping locks in moisture and creates a golden crust packed with flavor. Halibut is high in protein and omega-3 and omega-6 fatty acids, like other fish, but is also an excellent source of selenium, niacin, phosphorus magnesium, and vitamins B_6 and B_{12}. Including halibut in your diet can help decrease inflammation, support the thyroid, prevent cardiovascular disease, and regulate the metabolism.

4 (4-ounce) halibut fillets

Sea salt

Freshly ground black pepper

½ cup Traditional Hummus (page 188) or store-bought hummus

¼ cup whole-wheat panko breadcrumbs

1 tablespoon chopped fresh oregano

1. Preheat the oven to 400°F.

2. Lightly season the halibut with salt and pepper and place on a baking sheet. Spread the hummus on each fillet and sprinkle with the breadcrumbs.

3. Bake the fish until it flakes easily with a fork, about 15 minutes. Serve topped with oregano.

PER SERVING: *Calories: 193; Total fat: 3g; Saturated fat: 1g; Carbohydrates: 13g; Sugar: 1g; Fiber: 1g; Protein: 27g*

Moroccan Couscous Salad

SERVES 4 • DAIRY-FREE • MEAL IN ONE • VEGAN

PREP TIME:
20 MINUTES,
PLUS 2 HOURS
CHILLING TIME

COOK TIME:
10 MINUTES

Moroccan cuisine is a tasty mix of several different cuisines, such as Arabic, Berber, Mediterranean, and a smattering of European influence. Fresh produce, citrus, spices, nuts, dried fruit, and legumes all play a part in meal planning. The dried apricots featured in this salad are a common ingredient in salads, stews, and desserts. Apricots are very high in lycopene, an antioxidant that can inhibit the growth of cancer cells. This brightly colored fruit is also a great source of beta-carotene, fiber, iron, magnesium, and vitamins A, C, and E.

FOR THE DRESSING

¼ cup freshly squeezed lime juice

2 tablespoons olive oil

½ teaspoon ground cumin

¼ teaspoon ground coriander

Sea salt

Freshly ground black pepper

FOR THE SALAD

1 cup couscous

1 (15-ounce) can low-sodium lentils, rinsed and drained

2 cups finely chopped broccoli

2 large carrots, peeled and shredded

½ cup chopped dried apricots

¼ cup chopped pistachios

1 tablespoon chopped fresh mint

TO MAKE THE DRESSING

In a small bowl, whisk the lime juice, olive oil, cumin, and coriander until blended. Season with salt and pepper and set aside.

TO MAKE THE SALAD

1. In a pot, bring 1½ cups water to a boil. Stir the couscous into the boiling water and remove from the heat. Cover and let sit for 10 minutes. Fluff with a fork.

2. Transfer the couscous to a large bowl and add the lentils, broccoli, carrots, apricots, pistachios, mint, and dressing. Stir to combine, cover, and place in the refrigerator until chilled, about 2 hours. Serve.

SUBSTITUTION TIP: *Pistachios create texture and crunch but can be left out if nut allergies are an issue, in which case try sesame seeds, sunflower seeds, and delicious toasted chickpeas instead.*

PER SERVING: *Calories: 401; Total fat: 10g; Saturated fat: 1g; Carbohydrates: 64g; Sugar: 7g; Fiber: 13g; Protein: 17g*

North African Chicken Apricot Tagine

SERVES 4 • DAIRY-FREE • GLUTEN-FREE • MEAL IN ONE

PREP TIME:
10 MINUTES

COOK TIME:
50 MINUTES

Cauliflower provides bulk to this dish and soaks up all the delightful warm spices, such as ginger, cumin, and cinnamon. Cauliflower is a member of the cruciferous family and contains the beneficial indole-3-carbinol, or I3C, and the phytonutrient sulforaphane. This vegetable has great disease-fighting capabilities and can lower the incidence of breast tumors. Cauliflower also has a lot of vitamin C and folate, which are antioxidants and help the blood and immune systems work more effectively. Most often, you will see a white cauliflower, but many markets sell purple and orange varieties. The gorgeous leaves surrounding the white cauliflower can also be eaten after being steamed or blanched, and taste like cabbage.

2 tablespoons olive oil, divided

1 pound boneless skinless chicken breast, cut into 1-inch chunks

½ sweet onion, chopped

1 tablespoon minced garlic

2 teaspoons peeled grated fresh ginger

2 cups cauliflower florets

2 carrots, cut in half lengthwise and sliced

1 (15-ounce) can low-sodium diced tomatoes

¼ cup chopped dried apricots

1 teaspoon ground cumin

½ teaspoon ground cinnamon

Sea salt

1. Preheat the oven to 400°F.

2. In a large ovenproof skillet, heat 1 tablespoon of olive oil. Brown the chicken until golden, about 10 minutes total. Transfer to a plate and set aside.

3. Add the remaining 1 tablespoon of olive oil and sauté the onion, garlic, and ginger until softened, about 3 minutes. Add the cauliflower and carrots and sauté for 5 minutes more.

4. Stir in the chicken, tomatoes and their juices, apricots, cumin, and cinnamon. Cover and braise in the oven until the vegetables are tender and the chicken is cooked through, 20 to 25 minutes. Season with salt and serve.

SUBSTITUTION TIP: *Dried fruit is often found in North African cuisine. It adds a lovely sweetness to complex spicy recipes. You can use dates, raisins, and dried figs instead of apricots in the same amount.*

PER SERVING: *Calories: 252; Total fat: 9g; Saturated fat: 1g; Carbohydrates: 17g; Sugar: 10g; Fiber: 4g; Protein: 28g*

Baking Sheet Spicy Shrimp with Vegetables

SERVES 4 • DAIRY-FREE • GLUTEN-FREE • MEAL IN ONE • 30 MINUTES OR LESS

PREP TIME:
15 MINUTES

COOK TIME:
12 MINUTES

Shrimp cooks very quickly, so it is a great choice when you need a nutritious meal in a hurry. The colorful assortment of vegetables in this recipe cooks in the same time as the shellfish. Bok choy is not a traditional Mediterranean vegetable, but it shares the health benefits of the other members of the cabbage family and is mild enough to combine well with any ingredient.

1 pound shrimp, peeled and deveined

3 baby bok choy, quartered

10 asparagus spears, trimmed and halved

1 yellow zucchini, sliced

1 red bell pepper, cut into thin strips

1 sweet onion, thinly sliced

1 tablespoon olive oil

½ teaspoon smoked paprika

½ teaspoon chili powder

½ teaspoon garlic powder

½ teaspoon ground cumin

Juice of 1 lime

1. Preheat the oven to 400°F.

2. In a large bowl, toss together the shrimp, bok choy, asparagus, zucchini, bell pepper, onion, olive oil, paprika, chili powder, garlic powder, and cumin until well coated. Spread the shrimp and vegetables on a baking sheet.

3. Bake until the shrimp are cooked through and vegetables are tender, stirring a few times, 10 to 12 minutes. Squeeze the lime juice over the shrimp and vegetables. Serve.

PER SERVING: *Calories: 181; Total fat: 5g; Saturated fat: 1g; Carbohydrates: 11g; Sugar: 5g; Fiber: 4g; Protein: 27g*

Chickpea Veggie Burgers

SERVES 4 • DAIRY-FREE • VEGETARIAN

PREP TIME:
20 MINUTES,
PLUS 1 HOUR
CHILLING TIME

COOK TIME:
15 MINUTES

This burger might remind you of falafel, although it has a distinct golden color from the added turmeric and bright carrot shreds. Turmeric has an active agent called curcumin, which has anticancer and anti-inflammatory effects. Adding black pepper to the burger boosts the absorption rate of the curcumin by 1,000 times.

2 tablespoons olive oil, divided

½ sweet onion, chopped

½ carrot, shredded

1 celery stalk, chopped

1 teaspoon minced garlic

1 (15-ounce) can low-sodium chickpeas, drained and rinsed

1 large egg

¼ cup panko breadcrumbs

1 teaspoon ground cumin

¼ teaspoon turmeric

⅛ teaspoon freshly ground black pepper

1. In a large skillet, heat 1 tablespoon of olive oil over medium-high heat. Sauté the onion, carrot, celery, and garlic until softened, about 4 minutes.

2. Transfer the vegetables to a food processor and add the chickpeas, egg, breadcrumbs, cumin, turmeric, and pepper and pulse until the mixture is finely chopped and holds together when pressed. Divide the mixture to form 8 patties and chill in the refrigerator, covered, for 1 hour to firm up.

3. Heat the remaining 1 tablespoon of olive oil in a large skillet over medium heat. Cook the patties until golden on both sides, turning once, about 10 minutes total. Serve.

PER SERVING: *Calories: 266; Total fat: 10g; Saturated fat: 2g; Carbohydrates: 372g; Sugar: 1g; Fiber: 7g; Protein: 9g*

Barley Risotto with Sweet Potato and Spinach

SERVES 4 • MEAL IN ONE • VEGETARIAN

PREP TIME:
10 MINUTES, PLUS
SOAKING TIME

COOK TIME:
40 MINUTES

B arley is a nutty, chewy grain with a taste and texture that holds up well to earthy spinach, sweet potato, and a healthy amount of garlic. Any food that contains vitamin A, like sweet potato, is great for the skin, which is a barrier against all the toxins, viruses, and environmental threats in your life.

1 tablespoon olive oil

½ sweet onion, finely chopped

1 teaspoon minced garlic

1 cup pearl barley, soaked overnight, drained, and rinsed

2 sweet potatoes, peeled and cut into ¼-inch pieces

3 cups low-sodium vegetable stock

2 cups packed baby spinach

½ cup grated Parmesan cheese

1 tablespoon butter

Sea salt

Freshly ground black pepper

1. Preheat the oven to 400°F.

2. In a large ovenproof skillet, heat the olive oil over medium-high heat. Sauté the onion and garlic until softened, about 3 minutes.

3. Stir in the barley, sweet potatoes, and vegetable stock. Cover the skillet and transfer to the oven. Bake until the barley is tender and the liquid is absorbed, about 35 minutes.

4. Remove the skillet from the oven and stir in the spinach, Parmesan cheese, and butter. Season with salt and pepper and serve.

PER SERVING: *Calories: 342; Total fat: 10g; Saturated fat: 5g; Carbohydrates: 54g; Sugar: 4g; Fiber: 11g; Protein: 11g*

Tunisian Herb Chicken Skewers

SERVES 4 • DAIRY-FREE • GLUTEN-FREE

PREP TIME:
10 MINUTES,
PLUS 2 HOURS
MARINATING TIME

COOK TIME:
10 MINUTES

Skewers are a fun way of serving many ingredients, such as these spiced chicken beauties. Paprika is made from the ground pods of *Capsicum annuum* peppers. Many types of paprika are created from different pepper variations and drying processes, such as smoking or toasting. Paprika is rich in vitamin A, beta-carotene, potassium, copper, and iron. This spice can help prevent cancer and macular degeneration and support a healthy cardiovascular system.

¼ cup olive oil

¼ cup freshly squeezed lemon juice

1 tablespoon chopped fresh thyme

2 tablespoons smoked paprika

1 tablespoon minced garlic

1 tablespoon chopped fresh parsley

1 teaspoon ground cumin

1 pound boneless, skinless chicken breasts, cut into 1½-inch chunks

1. In a large bowl, stir together the olive oil, lemon juice, thyme, paprika, garlic, parsley, and cumin until well mixed. Add the chicken, stirring to coat, cover, and refrigerate 2 hours.

2. Preheat a grill to medium high. Soak 8 bamboo skewers in warm water.

3. Thread the chicken chunks onto soaked wooden skewers. Grill until the chicken is browned and cooked through, turning occasionally, 8 to 10 minutes. Serve.

COOKING TIP: *If you do not want to use skewers, leave the chicken breasts whole and pan-sear them in 1 tablespoon of olive oil over medium-high heat in a large skillet, after marinating. Then place them on a baking sheet and roast in a 400°F oven until cooked through and golden brown, 25 to 30 minutes total.*

PER SERVING: *Calories: 253; Total fat: 15g; Saturated fat: 2g; Carbohydrates: 4g; Sugar: 1g; Fiber: 2g; Protein: 27g*

Chicken Shawarma Bowls

SERVES 4 • GLUTEN-FREE • MEAL IN ONE

PREP TIME:
20 MINUTES,
PLUS 1 HOUR
MARINATING TIME

COOK TIME:
15 MINUTES

The foundation of shawarma is the blend of many spices balanced perfectly with just enough heat. Ginger and cayenne are spicy, and good for the circulatory system. Ginger warms the body and stimulates blood flow. It can also protect cardiovascular health by lowering cholesterol levels. Cayenne stimulates blood flow in several organs and systems and can also lower the fat levels in the blood.

1 pound boneless, skinless chicken breast, chopped

Juice of ½ lemon

½ teaspoon ground coriander

¼ teaspoon paprika

¼ teaspoon ground cumin

¼ teaspoon ground cinnamon

¼ teaspoon ground ginger

⅛ teaspoon ground cardamom

Pinch cayenne pepper

1 cup quinoa

2 cups water

1 tablespoon olive oil

1 cup canned low-sodium chickpeas, drained and rinsed

1 cup shredded spinach

2 tomatoes, chopped

½ English cucumber, chopped

¼ red onion, thinly sliced

½ cup Tzatziki Sauce (page 192)

2 tablespoons chopped fresh parsley

1. In a medium bowl, mix the chicken with the lemon juice, coriander, paprika, cumin, cinnamon, ginger, cardamom, and cayenne until very well coated. Cover the bowl and place in the refrigerator to mellow the flavors for 1 hour, stirring once.

2. While the chicken is marinating, rinse the quinoa under cold running water to remove its bitter flavor. In a small saucepan, combine the quinoa and water and bring to a boil over medium heat. Reduce the heat to low and simmer, uncovered, until the liquid is absorbed, 10 to 15 minutes.

3. While the quinoa is cooking, heat the olive oil in a large skillet over medium-high heat and sauté the chicken, stirring occasionally, until cooked through, about 15 minutes.

4. Divide the quinoa, chickpeas, and spinach between bowls. Divide the chicken between the bowls and top with tomatoes, cucumber, and onion. Spoon the tzatziki on top of each and garnish with parsley. Serve.

SUBSTITUTION TIP: *If you don't want to mix the plethora of spices to make your own shawarma blend, there are premade versions available in the spice section of your local grocery store. This can eliminate the need to have so many different spices on hand.*

PER SERVING: *Calories: 365; Total fat: 6g; Saturated fat: 1g; Carbohydrates: 38g; Sugar: 3g; Fiber: 7g; Protein: 38g*

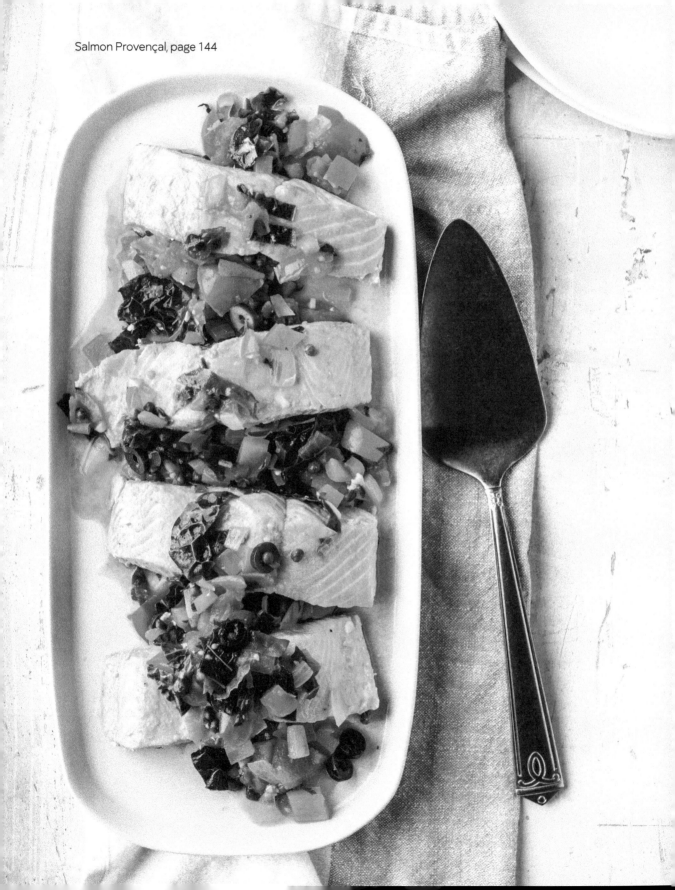

Salmon Provençal, page 144

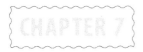

CHAPTER 7

After the Four-Week Plan

Congratulations! You should be extremely proud of yourself for getting through the first four weeks! It takes hard work and dedication to get as far as you did. It's no easy task. However, I do think it will get easier for you from here on out. Planning ahead and staying organized with your shopping lists will help you stay on track. And after four weeks of following the meal plans in this book, you are more than ready to go forth and plan your own Mediterranean diet–friendly meals and experiment with more Mediterranean flavors and recipes. This chapter will give you ideas for how to get creative with your meals and avoid falling off the wagon. But even if you do fall off the wagon once in a while, it's okay—just get back on, renew your dedication to achieving your health goals, and move forward.

PLANNING YOUR WEEK

Planning a weekly menu and creating a shopping list are key to setting yourself up for success on this diet. These steps will ensure you purchase only what you need and are able to easily make healthy meals all week long. I know it may take some getting used to initially, but I promise it will get much easier. The more organized you are at the beginning of the week, the healthier choices you will make during it.

Here are some tips for creating your menu and grocery list:

Create a recipe file. Keep a list of recipes you would like to try. Whether you file paper recipes from magazines and newspapers or you bookmark webpages online, create a place to store all the recipes you think you would like to make. Use this file as a reference when you are planning your menus.

See what you already have. Go through your panty, refrigerator, and freezer to assess your ingredients. Make a list and save money by incorporating these items in your weekly meal plans.

Keep a meal journal. Keeping track of everything will help you stay on goal. It is also great for looking back and planning future meals.

Plan around your life. When you are making a meal plan, be sure to plan for busy days in your schedule when you may not have as much time for cooking. Include several recipes that are quick and easy to prepare so that the plan will actually work with your life. Also, by looking at your schedule, you may see days that you will have no time to cook and you can plan on making extras of a meal in advance to serve on those no-cook nights.

Choose a shopping day and make a shopping list. You may find it easier to have success in meal preparation when your grocery shopping is planned very purposefully. Make a shopping list and pick a day to go shopping. There is also a blank meal plan at the back of the book you can photocopy and use.

Prep foods shortly after purchase. Do as much initial prep work as you can when you get home from the store. Wash lettuces and other greens. Chop hardier vegetables like broccoli and bell peppers for dishes later in the week. Grill or roast chicken to top salads. Store the prepped ingredients in glass or BPA-free plastic storage containers in the refrigerator to save time on meal prep throughout the week.

Make it fun. For a lot of people, having themed nights is an easy way to cut down on planning. If you make Tuesday "pita sandwiches night" and Friday "fish night," you have already taken some of the planning off your list. This may not work for all people, but especially if you have kids, this can be a fun way to get the whole family involved in mealtime.

MEDITERRANEAN MEALS FAST

Because we are always on the go, we often have little time to think about breakfast, let alone a healthy one. This section will give you some ideas for how to make quick Mediterranean meals, including breakfasts.

BREAKFAST BUILDER

Skipping breakfast is never a good idea. Some skip breakfast to try to cut calories, some are too busy during the morning rush, and others just don't feel hungry. But eating a good breakfast is an important part of a healthy lifestyle. This section will help you keep some breakfast food staples on hand to make eating even a rushed breakfast easy. The following three-column table emphasizes a healthy combination of proteins, fruit, and whole grains you can easily combine (and potentially mix and match):

WHOLE GRAIN	PROTEIN	FRUIT
Whole-grain muffin	1 boiled egg	Apple
¼ cup unsweetened granola	1 cup Greek yogurt	¼ cup berries
Whole-grain toast	1 tablespoon almond butter	Banana
Whole-grain toast	1 ounce fresh mozzarella	Tomato
1 cup cooked oatmeal	¼ cup raw almonds	¼ cup strawberries

Repurposing Ingredients

Save money and avoid wasting food by repurposing leftover ingredients to create flavorful new recipes. Here are a few tips to help you stretch the ingredients you have on hand and resist spending more money at the grocery store:

- If you have leftover frittata, stuff it into a whole-grain pita with some baby greens for a delicious lunch the next day.
- Use extra salad dressing for marinating protein. For example, use leftover Roasted Red Pepper Dressing (page 150) to marinate chicken overnight before baking or grilling.
- Take advantage of any leftover rice and couscous recipes to serve as a side with fish, chicken, or vegetables. You can even cook up extra to save for a quick Mediterranean grain bowl.
- If you buy green beans, peppers, onions, mushrooms, broccoli, squash, or spinach as side dishes for other meals, prep and store the excess in the refrigerator to easily throw into a quick frittata or egg scrambler.

MAKING A MEDITERRANEAN GRAIN BOWL

This section will help you make a Mediterranean diet–friendly bowl without a recipe, using what you have at the ready in your refrigerator. I recommend following this formula: whole grains + proteins + vegetables + garnishes + dressing.

Whole grains:

Choose from quinoa, spelt, whole-grain barley, bulgur wheat, brown rice, black rice, red rice, or wild rice.

Proteins:

Go plant-based with beans, lentils, chickpeas, edamame, baked tofu, or tempeh. Or if you prefer, use roasted chicken, leftover steak or fish, or even canned tuna or salmon.

Vegetables:

Prepare a batch of roasted veggies like Brussels sprouts, broccoli, cauliflower, or asparagus, but also add in chopped, shredded, or thinly sliced raw veggies, like red or green cabbage, radishes, carrots, and salad greens.

Garnishes:

These can include chopped tree nuts (walnuts, almonds, pistachios), peanuts, seeds (sunflower, pumpkin), avocado, olives, capers, marinated artichokes, fresh herbs, and cheese.

Dressing:

Make a simple olive oil dressing with lots of citrus, garlic, and spices.

DRESSING   +   GARNISHES

VEGETABLES   +   PROTEINS

WHOLE GRAINS

Tips for Eating Out

Eating out can be difficult for some, especially when options are limited. Here are a few tips for being mindful when you are eating out:

Decline the breadbasket. Ask the waiter not to bring the breadbasket to the table. Many people are really tempted by bread, and consuming it before a meal when you are hungry can easily bump your caloric intake way above where it should be. Besides, you'll actually enjoy your entrée without feeling full after a few bites.

Avoid anything fried. If you're unsure whether a dish is fried, don't be afraid to ask. Good choices are generally mixed salads, grilled vegetables, or broth-based soups.

Choose from poultry, fish, or vegetarian options. Beef dishes usually have higher fat and calorie content. If you are craving beef, look for leaner cuts like flank or sirloin steak, tenderloin, or filet mignon.

Be cautious of sauces. Sauces are sometimes oil-based or contain tons of butter. Ask for the sauce on the side to control how much you use or select a healthier sauce. Increasing awareness of food allergies and food sensitivities has led to the greater availability of healthy substitutes.

Plan a potluck with friends instead of eating out. You could ask your friends to come over for a potluck dinner. Have each person bring a dish or beverage of choice—you're saving on money and calories, without sacrificing your social life.

SUCCESS ISN'T A STRAIGHT LINE

Success isn't a straight line, and it's certainly not black and white. If you slip up, let me rephrase that, *when* you slip up, it's absolutely okay—it happens to all of us. Deviation from the diet doesn't mean you're a failure and that you can't be successful on the Mediterranean diet. It simply means you're human. We all mess up from time to time. So, don't be discouraged if you plateau, don't see results immediately, or overindulge in your favorite food. Put yourself back on track by reminding yourself of your goals, finding inspiration in motivational images and words, or talking to a family member, friend, or another supportive member of your community for a boost of confidence. Remember that the Mediterranean diet isn't a crash diet; it's a lifestyle change for achieving enduring health. And in order to succeed, you have to practice self-compassion—be kind to yourself.

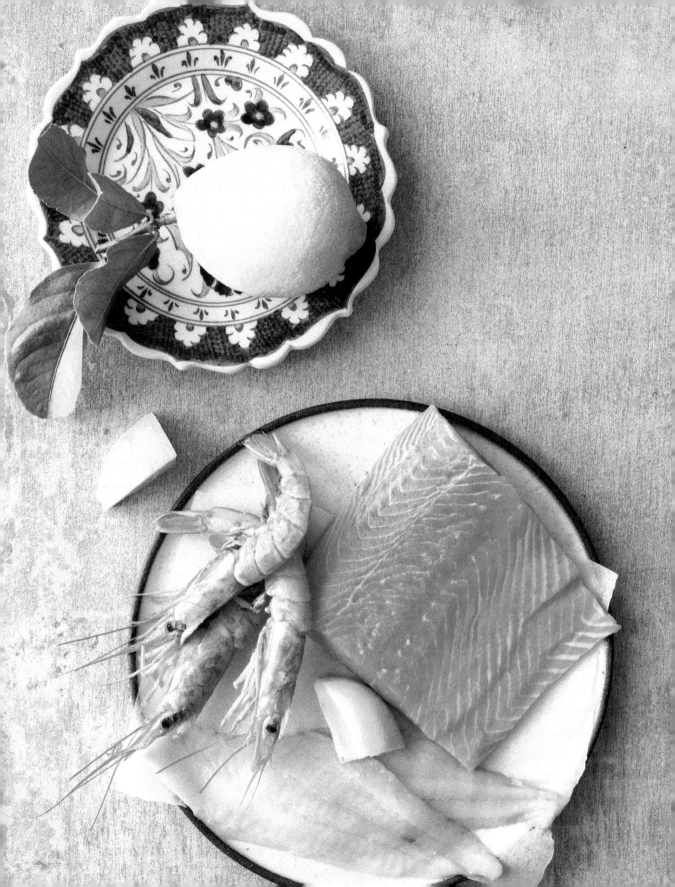

PART THREE

MEDITERRANEAN

RECIPES FOR LIFE

This section of the book provides you with additional recipes so you can continue cooking Mediterranean style and making your own meal plans. Preparing delicious and creative meals will give you more confidence as you continue on this path. And as you grow in confidence, I won't be surprised if you start experimenting with different ingredients and flavor combinations on your own one day!

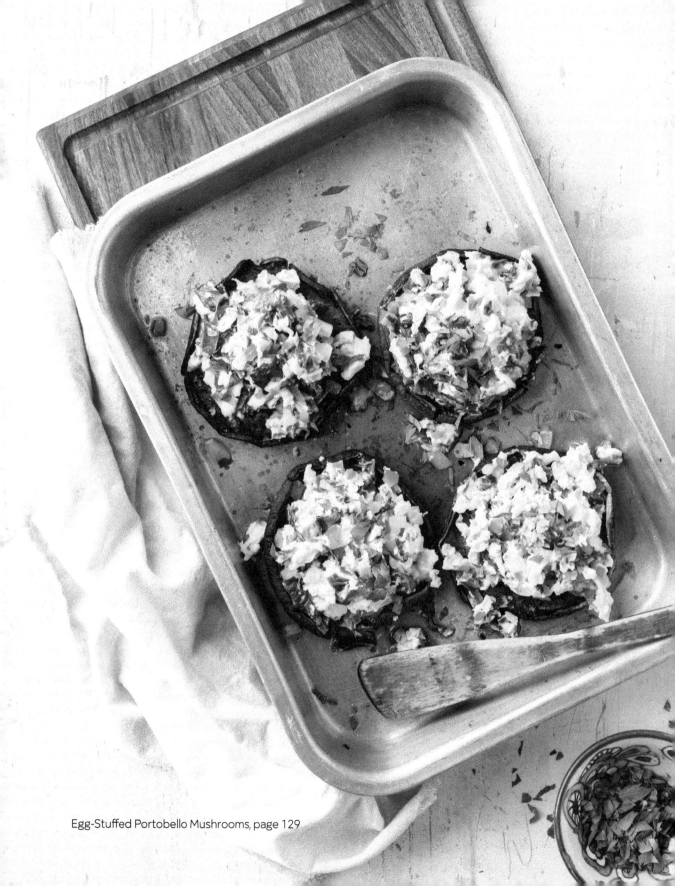

Egg-Stuffed Portobello Mushrooms, page 129

CHAPTER 8

Breakfast and Brunch

Oatmeal Bowls with Blackberries, Seeds, and Honey 124

Strawberry and Brown Rice Sunflower Seed Bowl 126

Cranberry-Pumpkin Smoothie 127

Quinoa-Walnut Pancakes 128

Egg-Stuffed Portobello Mushrooms 129

Greek Breakfast Tostadas 131

Tomato-Asparagus Omelets 132

Oatmeal Bowls with Blackberries, Seeds, and Honey

SERVES 4 • DAIRY-FREE • GLUTEN-FREE • MEAL IN ONE • VEGETARIAN • 30 MINUTES OR LESS

PREP TIME:
5 MINUTES

COOK TIME:
12 MINUTES

Porridge evokes visions of little gold-haired girls and bears for many people, and luckily, you will find this creamy porridge "just right" for any morning meal. Although mixed grain breakfast dishes are enjoyed in all Mediterranean countries, adding blackberries is most commonly done in the Andalusia region of Spain, where the sandy soil and warm climate are perfect for cultivating them. Blackberries are extremely rich in fiber, vitamins, minerals, antioxidants (such as ellagic acid), and anthocyanins, which give them their rich dark color.

2 cups water

¾ cup gluten-free rolled oats

¼ cup quinoa

2 tablespoons flaxseed

Pinch sea salt

½ cup unsweetened almond milk

½ teaspoon ground cinnamon

Pinch ground cloves

1 cup blackberries

¼ cup pumpkin seeds

2 tablespoons honey

1. In a medium saucepan, stir together the water, oats, quinoa, flaxseed, and salt and bring to a boil over medium-high heat. Cook, stirring constantly, for 5 minutes.

2. Reduce the heat to low and simmer until thick and creamy, 5 to 7 minutes.

3. Stir in the almond milk, cinnamon, and cloves.

4. Divide into bowls and top with the blackberries, pumpkin seeds, and honey. Serve.

SUBSTITUTION TIP: *Porridge can be a combination of any whole grains, such as freekeh, rye flakes, bulgur, barley, buckwheat groats, brown rice, steel-cut oats, and wheat berries. They do not have the same cooking times, so add the bigger, harder grains, such as wheat berries or barley, to the porridge already cooked.*

PER SERVING: *Calories: 253; Total fat: 10g; Saturated fat: 1g; Carbohydrates: 36g; Sugar: 11g; Fiber: 8g; Protein: 9g*

Strawberry and Brown Rice Sunflower Seed Bowl

SERVES 4 • DAIRY-FREE • GLUTEN-FREE • MEAL IN ONE • VEGETARIAN

PREP TIME:
5 MINUTES

COOK TIME:
45 MINUTES

Rice pudding does not have to be a dessert; it can also serve as a creamy, delectable breakfast. Strawberries are one of the most popular fruits in the world, and they add sweetness and color to this coconut-infused rice. Include strawberries in your diet whenever possible to help stabilize blood sugar, lower cholesterol and blood pressure, and improve digestion.

1 cup brown rice

1 cup water

1 cup light coconut milk

1 teaspoon pure vanilla extract

¼ teaspoon ground cinnamon

2 cups sliced strawberries

¼ cup sunflower seeds

¼ cup shredded unsweetened coconut

2 tablespoons honey

1. In a large saucepan, stir together the rice, water, coconut milk, vanilla, and cinnamon over medium-high heat.

2. Bring to a boil and then reduce the heat to low and simmer, covered, until the liquid is absorbed and the rice is tender, 35 to 40 minutes.

3. Remove from the heat and divide the rice between bowls. Top each bowl with strawberries, arranging them to cover half the rice. Add the sunflower seeds and coconut to the bowls so they each cover one-quarter of the rice.

4. Drizzle with honey and serve.

PER SERVING: *Calories: 299; Total fat: 8g; Saturated fat: 5g; Carbohydrates: 54g; Sugar: 13g; Fiber: 4g; Protein: 6g*

Cranberry-Pumpkin Smoothie

SERVES 2 • DAIRY-FREE • GLUTEN-FREE • MEAL IN ONE • VEGETARIAN • 30 MINUTES OR LESS

PREP TIME:
5 MINUTES

Cranberry and pumpkin are classic fall flavors, but you can enjoy this sunrise-hued smoothie year-round since canned and frozen pumpkin is readily available. Pure cranberry juice is very tart, so adjust the honey amount if you prefer a slightly sweeter result. Cranberries are extremely high in beta-carotene, folic acid, and vitamins B, C, and K. Their ruby juice is probably best known for treating and preventing urinary tract infections but can also reduce the risk of prostate cancer and kidney stones.

2 cups unsweetened almond milk

1 cup pure pumpkin purée

¼ cup gluten-free rolled oats

¼ cup pure cranberry juice (no sugar added)

1 tablespoon honey

¼ teaspoon ground cinnamon

Pinch ground nutmeg

1. In a blender, combine the almond milk, pumpkin, oats, cranberry juice, honey, cinnamon, and nutmeg and blend until smooth.

2. Pour into glasses and serve immediately.

SUBSTITUTION TIP: *Roasted or boiled mashed pumpkin can be used in place of canned pumpkin purée. If you are using the canned product, stay away from pie filling, which has extra sugar and spices that you do not need in your smoothie.*

PER SERVING: *Calories: 190; Total fat: 7g; Saturated fat: 0g; Carbohydrates: 26g; Sugar: 12g; Fiber: 5g; Protein: 4g*

Quinoa-Walnut Pancakes

SERVES 4 • DAIRY-FREE • MEAL IN ONE • VEGETARIAN • 30 MINUTES OR LESS

PREP TIME:
10 MINUTES

COOK TIME:
15 MINUTES

Almond milk is a popular choice for many people who do not consume dairy products or soy. Since almond milk contains only 60 calories per cup with no saturated fat, it is a healthy choice for weight loss. Almond milk is also low in carbs, which means it does not negatively impact blood sugar.

¾ cup whole-wheat flour

¼ cup ground walnuts

2 teaspoons baking powder

¼ teaspoon ground cinnamon

1 cup cooked quinoa

½ cup unsweetened almond milk

2 tablespoons honey

2 large eggs

2 teaspoons pure vanilla extract

Nonstick olive oil cooking spray

1. In a large bowl, stir together the flour, ground walnuts, baking powder, and cinnamon.

2. In a medium bowl, whisk together the quinoa, almond milk, honey, eggs, and vanilla until well blended. Add the quinoa mixture to the flour mixture and stir until mixed.

3. Heat a large skillet over medium heat and spray with cooking spray.

4. Scoop about ¼ cup of batter per pancake into the skillet, making about 4 pancakes per batch, and cook until puffed up and browned on the bottom, about 3 minutes. Flip and cook for about 2 minutes more, until browned. Transfer to a plate and repeat with remaining batter. Serve with your favorite toppings.

PER SERVING: *Calories: 271; Total fat: 9g; Saturated fat: 1g; Carbohydrates: 39g; Sugar: 9g; Fiber: 3g; Protein: 10g*

Egg-Stuffed Portobello Mushrooms

SERVES 4 • DAIRY-FREE • GLUTEN-FREE • MEAL IN ONE • VEGETARIAN • 30 MINUTES OR LESS

PREP TIME:
10 MINUTES

COOK TIME:
12 MINUTES

Portobello mushrooms are native to Italy and are featured in many Italian recipes. The large size and meaty texture of this fungus make it a natural container. Swiss chard works beautifully as part of a filling, especially if you look for smaller leaves, which have no bitter taste. This pretty, dark leafy green comes with different-color stalks—white, yellow, green, orange, and deep red—and contains almost every nutrient possible. Swiss chard boosts immunity, stabilizes blood sugar, supports healthy hair and skin, and reduces the risk of cancer, osteoporosis, cataracts, and macular degeneration.

4 large Portobello mushrooms

2 tablespoons olive oil, divided

Sea salt

Freshly ground black pepper

1 sweet onion, chopped

½ red bell pepper, finely chopped

1 teaspoon minced garlic

1 cup shredded Swiss chard

6 large eggs, beaten

1 tablespoon chopped fresh parsley

1. Preheat the oven to 425°F.

2. Remove the stems and scoop the black gills out of the mushrooms, creating a deep well. Rub the mushrooms with 1 tablespoon of olive oil and season with salt and pepper.

3. Place the mushrooms gill-side up on a baking sheet and roast until the mushrooms are tender, about 10 minutes.

4. While the mushrooms are baking, heat the remaining 1 tablespoon of olive oil in a large skillet and sauté the onion, bell pepper, and garlic on medium heat until softened, about 4 minutes.

Continued >

5. Add the chard and sauté until wilted, about 4 minutes. Stir in the eggs and scramble for about 4 minutes, until cooked through but still moist.

6. Spoon the eggs into the mushrooms and sprinkle with parsley. Serve.

INGREDIENT TIP: *Portobello mushrooms should be dry, both top and gills. You can chop the gills up along with any scooped-out flesh and add it to the egg filling, but the black gills will tint the eggs an unappetizing gray.*

PER SERVING: *Calories: 206; Total fat: 15g; Saturated fat: 3g; Carbohydrates: 8g; Sugar: 3g; Fiber: 2g; Protein: 13g*

Greek Breakfast Tostadas

SERVES 4 • GLUTEN-FREE • MEAL IN ONE • VEGETARIAN • 30 MINUTES OR LESS

PREP TIME:
15 MINUTES

COOK TIME:
10 MINUTES

You will be reminded of pizza when you see this crunchy egg and vegetable–topped round—it even has a lovely herb and cheese garnish. Mozzarella is very high in protein, calcium, and phosphorus, so it supports healthy bones and teeth.

4 tostadas

½ cup Traditional Hummus (page 188) or store-bought hummus

½ cup chopped sun-dried tomatoes

1 tablespoon olive oil

2 shallots, chopped

1 teaspoon minced garlic

8 large eggs, beaten

½ cup chopped marinated artichoke hearts

¼ cup chopped fresh basil

¼ cup shredded fresh mozzarella

1. Spread each tostada with the hummus and sprinkle with sun-dried tomatoes. Set aside.

2. In a large skillet, heat the olive oil over medium-high heat. Sauté the shallots and garlic until softened, about 3 minutes.

3. Add the eggs to the skillet and scramble until cooked through but still moist, about 4 minutes.

4. Stir in the artichoke hearts, basil, and mozzarella and scramble for 1 minute more. Top the tostadas with the egg mixture and serve.

SUBSTITUTION TIP: *Can't find premade tostadas in your local store? Make your own by baking corn tortillas brushed with olive oil in a 400°F oven for about 5 minutes per side. Cool and top.*

PER SERVING: *Calories: 334; Total fat: 19g; Saturated fat: 5g; Carbohydrates: 25g; Sugar: 5g; Fiber: 5g; Protein: 19g*

Tomato-Asparagus Omelets

SERVES 4 • DAIRY-FREE • GLUTEN-FREE • MEAL IN ONE • VEGETARIAN • 30 MINUTES OR LESS

PREP TIME:
10 MINUTES

COOK TIME:
20 MINUTES

There are many ways to flavor egg dishes, including herbs, spices, vegetables, and pungent alliums. Scallions are sometimes overlooked because they seem more like a garnish. They can have an almost sweet taste if the stalks are tender and young. Scallions are a stellar source of many vitamins, such as A, B, C, and K.

2 tablespoons olive oil, divided

12 asparagus spears, trimmed and cut into 2-inch pieces

1 cup shredded spinach

1 cup halved cherry tomatoes

1 scallion, both white and green parts, thinly sliced on the bias

8 large eggs

1 teaspoon chopped fresh basil

1 teaspoon chopped fresh parsley

Sea salt

Freshly ground black pepper

1. In a medium skillet, heat 2 teaspoons of olive oil over medium-high heat.

2. Sauté the asparagus, spinach, tomatoes, and scallion until tender, about 5 minutes. Remove from the skillet and set aside.

3. In a medium bowl, beat the eggs with the basil and parsley. Season lightly with salt and pepper.

4. Wipe the skillet out and add 2 teaspoons of olive oil. Pour half of the egg mixture into the skillet and let cook, without stirring, until edges are set. Using a spatula, lift the edges and let the uncooked eggs flow underneath. Repeat this process until the eggs are just cooked through, about 4 minutes.

5. Spoon half of the asparagus mixture on half of the omelet and flip the other side of the omelet over the filling. Transfer the omelet to a plate.

6. Repeat steps 4 and 5 with the remaining egg mixture and asparagus mixture to make another omelet.

7. Cut the omelets in half and serve.

SUBSTITUTION TIP: *If you have the time, use clarified butter instead of olive oil for your omelets. To make your own clarified butter (or ghee), place 2 cups of diced unsalted butter in a glass measuring cup and microwave on high for about 1½ minutes, until melted. Let stand for 1 to 2 minutes, until slightly cooled and the milk solids have settled on the bottom. Scoop out the foamy top layer. Spoon the clear layer into a container, discarding the milky liquid at the bottom. Store in a sealed container in the refrigerator for up to 6 months.*

PER SERVING: *Calories: 229; Total fat: 17g; Saturated fat: 4g; Carbohydrates: 6g; Sugar: 3g; Fiber: 2g; Protein: 15g*

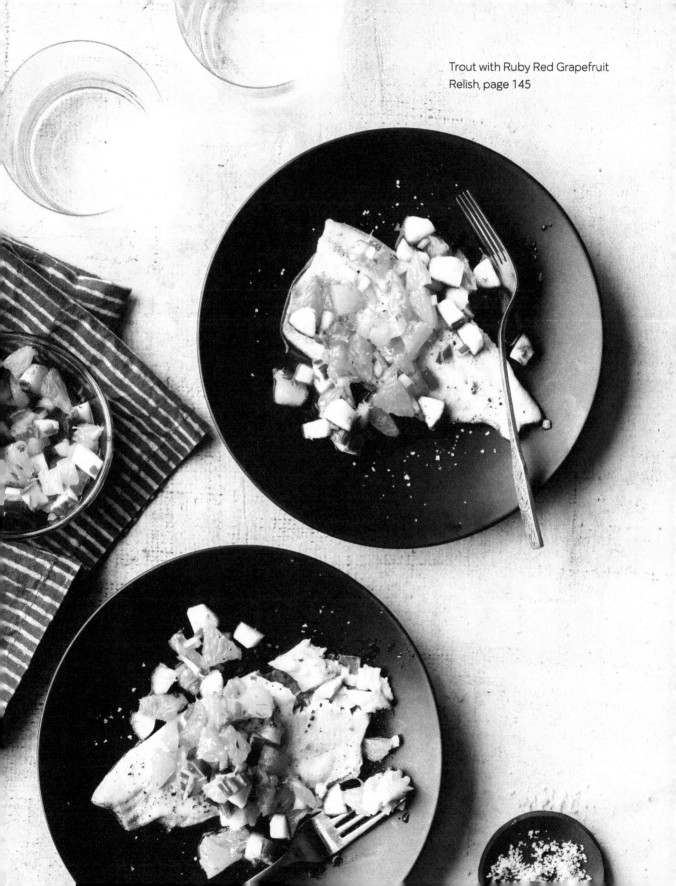

Trout with Ruby Red Grapefruit Relish, page 145

CHAPTER 9

Fish and Shellfish

Tomato and Wine-Steamed Mussels 136

Citrus-Herb Scallops 137

Spicy Broccoli-Shrimp Farfalle 138

Whole Baked Trout with Lemon and Herbs 140

Skillet Cod with Fresh Tomato Salsa 141

Broiled Flounder with Nectarine and White Bean Salsa 142

Baked Sardine Patties 143

Salmon Provençal 144

Trout with Ruby Red Grapefruit Relish 145

Tomato and Wine-Steamed Mussels

SERVES 4 • DAIRY-FREE • GLUTEN-FREE • MEAL IN ONE • 30 MINUTES OR LESS

PREP TIME:
10 MINUTES

COOK TIME:
15 MINUTES

Mussels are an incredibly flavorful, inexpensive ingredient that can be cooked quickly and served simply with a sauce or over whole-wheat pasta. Frozen mussels are a perfectly acceptable replacement for fresh ones. Thaw them, and then add them to the pot after bringing the other ingredients to a boil and simmer for 3 to 4 minutes.

1 tablespoon olive oil

1 sweet onion, chopped

1 tablespoon minced garlic

⅛ teaspoon red pepper flakes

4 tomatoes, chopped

¼ cup low-sodium fish or chicken stock

¼ cup dry white wine

3 pounds mussels, cleaned and rinsed

Juice and zest of 1 lemon

¼ cup pitted, sliced Kalamata olives

3 tablespoons chopped fresh parsley

Sea salt

Freshly ground black pepper

1. In a large saucepan, heat the olive oil over medium-high heat. Sauté the onion, garlic, and red pepper flakes until softened, about 3 minutes. Stir in the tomatoes, stock, and wine and bring to a boil.

2. Add the mussels to the saucepan and cover. Steam until the mussels are opened, 6 to 7 minutes. Remove from the heat and discard any unopened shells.

3. Stir in the lemon juice, lemon zest, olives, and parsley. Season with salt and pepper and serve.

PER SERVING: *Calories: 162; Total fat: 7g; Saturated fat: 1g; Carbohydrates: 12g; Sugar: 5g; Fiber: 3g; Protein: 12g*

Citrus-Herb Scallops

SERVES 4 • DAIRY-FREE • GLUTEN-FREE • 30 MINUTES OR LESS

PREP TIME:
10 MINUTES

COOK TIME:
4 MINUTES

Scallops are best eaten fresh, which means enjoying them between October and March, although you can get outstanding-quality frozen products. Scallops are often considered unhealthy because they are often served with calorie- and fat-laden sauces, but this simple, fresh preparation allows the scallop to shine through. Scallops are a great source of protein, potassium, and magnesium.

1 pound sea scallops

Sea salt

Freshly ground black pepper

2 tablespoons olive oil

Juice of 1 lime

Pinch red pepper flakes

1 tablespoon chopped fresh cilantro

1. Season the scallops lightly with salt and pepper.

2. In a large skillet, heat the olive oil over medium-high heat. Add the scallops to the skillet, making sure they do not touch one another.

3. Sear on both sides, turning once, for a total of about 3 minutes. Add the lime juice and red pepper flakes to the skillet and toss the scallops in the juice. Serve topped with cilantro.

INGREDIENT TIP: *Fresh scallops are in season from late fall through winter, so that is the best time to make this special dish. Look for drier scallops, not stored in a milky liquid called sodium triphosphate. This additive causes the scallops to soak up water, which means you are paying for water weight and your scallops will have less flavor.*

PER SERVING: *Calories: 160; Total fat: 8g; Saturated fat: 1g; Carbohydrates: 3g; Sugar: 0g; Fiber: 0g; Protein: 19g*

Spicy Broccoli-Shrimp Farfalle

SERVES 4 • DAIRY-FREE • MEAL IN ONE

PREP TIME:
15 MINUTES

COOK TIME:
20 MINUTES

Pasta is a complete meal, needing no other accents beyond a glass of nice wine or olive oil–slathered crusty whole-grain bread. Broccoli is very well known for its cancer-fighting abilities, so much so that the Hippocrates Institute recommends daily doses of it to prevent cancer. This cruciferous vegetable is an outstanding source of calcium, beta-carotene, vitamins A and B, indoles, iron, and essential amino acids including arginine, leucine, lysine, and valine. Along with being a powerful cancer fighter, broccoli reduces the risk of heart disease, stroke, and cataracts, supports healthy bones, and boosts the immune system.

4 | 8 ounces dry whole-wheat farfalle

1 | 2 tablespoons olive oil, divided

1/2 | 1 pound shrimp, peeled and deveined

2 | 4 cups small broccoli florets

1/2 | 1 yellow bell pepper, chopped

1 | 2 teaspoons minced garlic

Pinch red pepper flakes

1/2 | 1 cup halved cherry tomatoes

1/2 | Juice and zest from 1 lemon

Sea salt

Freshly ground black pepper

1/2 | 1 tablespoon chopped fresh parsley

1. Bring a large pot of water to a boil and cook the pasta according to the package instructions until al dente. Drain.

2. While the pasta is cooking, in a large skillet, heat 1 tablespoon of olive oil. Sauté the shrimp until they are just cooked through, 4 to 5 minutes. Remove the shrimp with a slotted spoon, transfer to a plate, and set aside.

3. Add the remaining 1 tablespoon of olive oil to the skillet and add the broccoli, bell pepper, garlic, and red pepper flakes. Sauté until the vegetables are crisp-tender, 6 to 7 minutes.

4. Stir in the cherry tomatoes, lemon juice, and lemon zest and cook until the tomatoes soften, about 3 minutes more; season with salt and pepper. Add the shrimp and pasta to the skillet, tossing to combine. Serve topped with parsley.

INGREDIENT TIP: *Scrub the outside of the lemon with a brush before zesting to remove any contaminants and the thin layer of wax that is applied to protect the fruit during transport. Organic lemons do not have the waxy layer, but should still be washed well.*

PER SERVING: *Calories: 388; Total fat: 10g; Saturated fat: 1g; Carbohydrates: 45g; Sugar: 6g; Fiber: 8g; Protein: 29g*

Whole Baked Trout with Lemon and Herbs

SERVES 4 • DAIRY-FREE • GLUTEN-FREE • MEAL IN ONE • 30 MINUTES OR LESS

PREP TIME:
10 MINUTES

COOK TIME:
20 MINUTES

Tender, fragrant baked whole fish festooned with herbs on serving platters in the middle of the table is a common sight in many North African and Mediterranean countries. Stuffing the cavity of the cleaned fish with herbs, vegetables, and citrus fruit is an effective way to infuse the fish with flavor.

1 tablespoon olive oil, divided

2 (8-ounce) whole trout, cleaned

Sea salt

Freshly ground black pepper

1 lemon, thinly sliced into about 6 pieces

1 tablespoon finely chopped fresh dill

1 tablespoon chopped fresh parsley

½ cup low-sodium fish stock or chicken stock

1. Preheat the oven to 400°F.

2. Lightly grease a 9-by-13-inch baking dish with 1 teaspoon of olive oil.

3. Rinse the trout, pat dry with paper towels, and coat with the remaining 2 teaspoons of olive oil. Season with salt and pepper.

4. Stuff the interior of the trout with the lemon slices, dill, and parsley and place into the prepared baking dish. Bake the fish for 10 minutes, then add the fish stock to the dish.

5. Continue to bake until the fish flakes easily with a fork, about 10 minutes. Serve.

PER SERVING: *Calories: 194; Total fat: 10g; Saturated fat: 2g; Carbohydrates: 1g; Sugar: 0g; Fiber: 0g; Protein: 25g*

Skillet Cod with Fresh Tomato Salsa

SERVES 4 • DAIRY-FREE • GLUTEN-FREE • 30 MINUTES OR LESS

PREP TIME:
20 MINUTES

COOK TIME:
8 MINUTES

Cod is a popular fish in European countries along the Mediterranean because of its mild taste and low mercury contamination. Like other fish, cod is a good source of omega-3 and omega-6 fatty acids, protein, iron, iodine, selenium, and zinc. If available, heirloom tomatoes make for an even prettier dish.

3 tomatoes, finely chopped

1 green bell pepper, finely chopped

¼ red onion, finely chopped

¼ cup pitted, chopped green olives

2 tablespoons white wine vinegar

1 tablespoon chopped fresh basil

½ teaspoon minced garlic

4 (4-ounce) cod fillets

Sea salt

Freshly ground black pepper

1 tablespoon olive oil

1. In a small bowl, stir together the tomatoes, bell pepper, onion, olives, vinegar, basil, and garlic until well mixed. Set aside.

2. Season the fish with salt and pepper.

3. In a large skillet, heat the olive oil over medium-high heat. Pan-fry the fish, turning once, until it is just cooked through, about 4 minutes per side.

4. Transfer to serving plates and top with a generous scoop of tomato salsa.

PER SERVING: *Calories: 181; Total fat: 7g; Saturated fat: 1g; Carbohydrates: 9g; Sugar: 4g; Fiber: 3g; Protein: 22g*

Broiled Flounder with Nectarine and White Bean Salsa

SERVES 4 • DAIRY-FREE • GLUTEN-FREE • 30 MINUTES OR LESS

PREP TIME:
20 MINUTES

COOK TIME:
8 MINUTES

This fish, bean, and fruit dish could be a poster meal for the Mediterranean diet. Nectarines are high in potassium, beta-carotene, pectin, calcium, iron, B vitamins, and vitamins A, C, and K. They are good for the cardiovascular system and reduce the risk of certain cancers.

2 nectarines, pitted and chopped

1 (15-ounce) can low-sodium cannellini beans, rinsed and drained

1 red bell pepper, chopped

1 scallion, both white and green parts, chopped

2 tablespoons chopped fresh cilantro

2 tablespoons freshly squeezed lime juice

4 (4-ounce) flounder fillets

1 teaspoon smoked paprika

Sea salt

Freshly ground black pepper

1. Preheat the oven to broil.

2. In a medium bowl, combine the nectarines, beans, bell pepper, scallion, cilantro, and lime juice.

3. Season the fish with paprika, salt, and pepper.

4. Place the fish on a baking sheet and broil, turning once, until just cooked through, about 8 minutes total. Serve the fish topped with the salsa.

INGREDIENT TIP: *Flounder is a type of bottom-dwelling flatfish; you can substitute fish labeled fluke, common dab, plaice, gray sole, petrale sole, or lemon sole.*

PER SERVING: *Calories: 259; Total fat: 8g; Saturated fat: 1g; Carbohydrates: 23g; Sugar: 8g; Fiber: 7g; Protein: 26g*

Baked Sardine Patties

SERVES 4 • DAIRY-FREE

PREP TIME:
15 MINUTES,
PLUS 1 HOUR
CHILLING TIME

COOK TIME:
20 MINUTES

These tasty sardine patties are such a treat! Sardines are incredibly nutritious and are an inexpensive ingredient, especially when purchased in convenient cans. They are an excellent source of two essential fats, linoleic acid (omega-6) and alpha-linolenic acid (omega-3).

3 (5-ounce) cans boneless, water-packed sardines, drained

¾ cup panko breadcrumbs

2 large eggs

1 scallion, both white and green parts, finely chopped

2 teaspoons freshly squeezed lemon juice

2 teaspoons chopped fresh dill

Sea salt

Freshly ground black pepper

1 tablespoon olive oil

1. In a medium bowl, mash the sardines with a fork. Add the breadcrumbs, eggs, scallion, lemon juice, and dill and stir until the mixture holds together when pressed. Add more lemon juice if too dry and more breadcrumbs if too wet. Season with salt and pepper.

2. Form the mixture into 12 patties, about ½-inch thick. Place them in the refrigerator, covered, for about 1 hour to firm up.

3. Preheat the oven to 350°F.

4. Transfer the patties to a baking sheet and brush them on both sides with the olive oil. Bake, turning once, until golden brown, 18 to 20 minutes total. Serve.

SUBSTITUTION TIP: *Use the same amount of ground almonds in place of the panko for an interesting, rich flavor and a gluten-free meal.*

PER SERVING: *Calories: 197; Total fat: 9g; Saturated fat: 2g; Carbohydrates: 19g; Sugar: 0g; Fiber: 1g; Protein: 12g*

Salmon Provençal

SERVES 4 • DAIRY-FREE • GLUTEN-FREE

PREP TIME:
15 MINUTES

COOK TIME:
25 MINUTES

Provençal cuisine takes advantage of the warm Mediterranean climate, bountiful produce, and fresh seafood from the coast. The healthy ingredients in this recipe positively impact your entire body. Salmon is rich in the essential fatty acids required for healthy muscles as well as the protein that can accelerate muscle recovery rates.

1 tablespoon olive oil

1 red bell pepper, chopped

½ sweet onion, chopped

2 teaspoons minced garlic

3 large tomatoes, chopped

1 cup shredded kale

¼ cup dry white wine

¼ cup pitted, sliced black olives

2 tablespoons capers

1 teaspoon chopped fresh thyme

1 teaspoon chopped fresh parsley

4 (4-ounce) salmon fillets

1. Preheat the oven to 400°F.

2. In a large ovenproof skillet, heat the olive oil over medium-high heat. Sauté the bell pepper, onion, and garlic until softened, about 4 minutes.

3. Add the tomatoes, kale, and wine and bring the mixture to a boil. Reduce the heat to low and simmer until the sauce thickens slightly, about 5 minutes.

4. Stir in the olives, capers, thyme, and parsley. Nestle the salmon fillets in the sauce, cover, and braise in the oven until the fish flakes easily with a fork, 15 to 18 minutes. Remove from the oven and serve the salmon topped with the sauce.

PER SERVING: *Calories: 314; Total fat: 18g; Saturated fat: 3g; Carbohydrates: 11g; Sugar: 6g; Fiber: 3g; Protein: 26g*

Trout with Ruby Red Grapefruit Relish

SERVES 4 • DAIRY-FREE • GLUTEN-FREE • 30 MINUTES OR LESS

PREP TIME:
15 MINUTES

COOK TIME:
15 MINUTES

It is no surprise that seafood plays such a huge role in the Italian diet when you consider that almost every region in Italy has a coastline stretch on the Mediterranean providing heaps of seafood plus wonderful freshwater fish like trout. Peperoncini add a potent heat to the tart, colorful relish, and they contain even more vitamin C than the citrus fruit, as well as vitamins A and B, fiber, and potassium.

1 ruby red grapefruit, peeled, sectioned, and chopped

1 large navel orange, peeled, sectioned, and chopped

¼ English cucumber, chopped

2 tablespoons chopped red onion

1 tablespoon minced or grated lime zest

1 teaspoon minced fresh or canned peperoncino

1 teaspoon chopped fresh thyme

4 (4-ounce) trout fillets

Sea salt

Freshly ground black pepper

1 tablespoon olive oil

1. Preheat the oven to 400°F.

2. In a medium bowl, stir together the grapefruit, orange, cucumber, onion, lime zest, peperoncino, and thyme. Cover the relish with plastic wrap and set aside in the refrigerator.

3. Season the trout lightly with salt and pepper and place on a baking sheet.

4. Brush the fish with olive oil and roast in the oven until it flakes easily with a fork, about 15 minutes. Serve topped with the chilled relish.

PER SERVING: *Calories: 178; Total fat: 6g; Saturated fat: 1g; Carbohydrates: 10g; Sugar: 7g; Fiber: 2g; Protein: 25g*

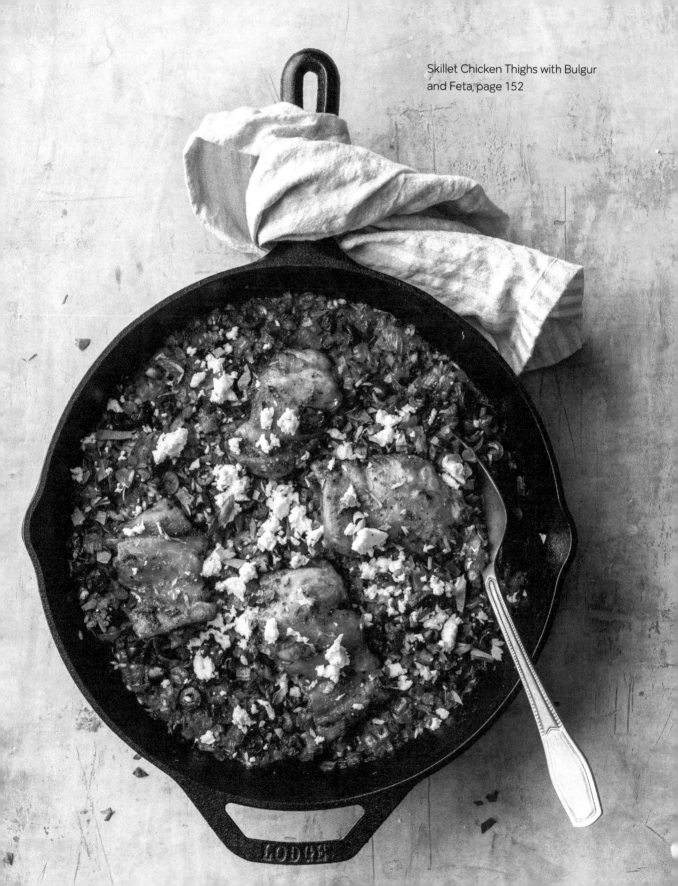

Skillet Chicken Thighs with Bulgur and Feta, page 152

CHAPTER 10

Poultry and Lean Meat

Pan-Fried Chicken with Roasted Squash Salsa 148

Chicken-Lentil Bowl with Roasted Red Pepper Dressing 150

Skillet Chicken Thighs with Bulgur and Feta 152

Turkey-Tomato Ragù 154

Chickpea-Turkey Stew with Spinach 155

Classic Pork Tenderloin Marsala 157

Rosemary-Citrus Roasted Pork Tenderloin 159

Chili-Spiced Lamb Chops 160

Greek Herbed Beef Meatballs 161

Pan-Fried Chicken with Roasted Squash Salsa

SERVES 4 • DAIRY-FREE • GLUTEN-FREE

PREP TIME:
15 MINUTES

COOK TIME:
20 MINUTES

This dish seems like it should be served in the autumn, with its golden topping and warm spice-infused scent. However, since squash is available year-round, you can create this recipe whenever you need a simple but glorious meal. The color of the squash is an indicator that the fruit is high in beta-carotene, and it is also an excellent source of potassium and vitamins A, B_6, C, and E. Including sunny-hued squash regularly in your diet can help stabilize blood sugar, reduce the risk of heart disease and cancer, and protect against diabetes and macular degeneration.

½ butternut squash, peeled and cut into ¼-inch cubes

1 tablespoon olive oil, divided

1 teaspoon ground cinnamon

Sea salt

Freshly ground black pepper

1 pear, cored and chopped

1 scallion, both white and green parts, thinly sliced on the bias

1 tablespoon freshly squeezed lemon juice

4 (3-ounce) boneless, skinless chicken breasts, pounded to 1-inch thick

1. Preheat the oven to 400°F. Line a baking sheet with aluminum foil and set aside.

2. In a medium bowl, toss the squash with 1 teaspoon of olive oil and the cinnamon. Season the squash lightly with salt and pepper.

3. Spread the squash on the baking sheet and bake until tender and lightly caramelized, about 15 minutes. Transfer from the baking sheet to a medium bowl and let cool for about 10 minutes.

4. Stir in the pear, scallion, and lemon juice, toss to combine, and set aside.

5. While the squash is baking, in a large skillet, heat the remaining 2 teaspoons of olive oil over medium-high heat.

6. Season the chicken breast with salt and pepper and pan-fry until golden and cooked through, turning once, about 15 minutes. Serve the chicken with the roasted squash salsa.

COOKING TIP: *Finding small chicken breasts, 3 ounces each, might be a challenge in most grocery stores. Pick up 6-ounce breasts instead and cut them in half horizontally before pounding them between two pieces of plastic wrap.*

PER SERVING: *Calories: 189; Total fat: 5g; Saturated fat: 1g; Carbohydrates: 18g; Sugar: 6g; Fiber: 3g; Protein: 21g*

Chicken-Lentil Bowl with Roasted Red Pepper Dressing

SERVES 4 • DAIRY-FREE • GLUTEN-FREE • MEAL IN ONE • 30 MINUTES OR LESS

PREP TIME:
25 MINUTES

The variations possible when putting together a bowl are unlimited when using different proteins, legumes, nuts, vegetables, fruits, dressings, herbs, and dark leafy greens. Kale is a staple food in the Mediterranean diet because it is packed with nutrients and has so many positive impacts on the body. One issue many people contend with is anemia, which can be caused by iron deficiency and lack of folic acid. Dark leafy greens are very rich in iron and vitamin C (which increases the absorption of iron), as well as folic acid, so regular consumption of delicious dishes like this one can be an effective preventive measure for diet-related anemia.

FOR THE DRESSING

½ cup store-bought or homemade roasted red peppers

¼ cup olive oil

2 tablespoons balsamic vinegar

½ teaspoon minced garlic

Sea salt

Freshly ground black pepper

FOR THE LENTIL BOWL

2 (15-ounce) cans low-sodium lentils

2 cups chopped store-bought rotisserie chicken

2 cups halved cherry tomatoes

½ English cucumber, chopped

1 cup shredded kale

1 cup chopped marinated artichoke hearts

2 tablespoons chopped fresh basil

In a blender, combine the roasted red peppers, olive oil, balsamic vinegar, and garlic and pulse until finely chopped and smooth. Season with salt and pepper and set aside.

1. In a large bowl, toss together the lentils, chicken, and cherry tomatoes until mixed.

2. Divide the lentil mixture between bowls and top them evenly with cucumber, kale, artichoke hearts, and basil. Drizzle the roasted red pepper dressing over the bowls and serve.

COOKING TIP: *Cooked chicken breasts are a convenient ingredient to have on hand for salads, wraps, soups, and bowls when eating healthy. Prepare 8 to 10 breasts at the beginning of the week by baking them in a 375°F oven for 20 to 25 minutes, cooling, and storing them either in individual sealed plastic bags or in portions of 2 or 4. Cooked chicken will keep for 5 days in the refrigerator.*

PER SERVING: *Calories: 504; Total fat: 18g; Saturated fat: 3g; Carbohydrates: 48g; Sugar: 6g; Fiber: 18g; Protein: 40g*

Skillet Chicken Thighs with Bulgur and Feta

SERVES 4 • MEAL IN ONE

PREP TIME:
10 MINUTES

COOK TIME:
40 MINUTES

One-pot cooking can be a busy person's lifeline, especially if you have a family to feed. Plain chicken and rice are upgraded to juicy lemony thighs and garlic-flavored bulgur. Bulgur combined with a healthy amount of dark green parsley adds vitamin C and E to your diet. These vitamins are powerful antioxidants that help eliminate free radicals in the body. Free radicals are considered a contributing factor in many diseases, such as cancer and Alzheimer's.

4 (3-ounce) boneless skinless chicken thighs

Sea salt

Freshly ground black pepper

Zest of 1 lemon

2 tablespoons olive oil

1 sweet onion, chopped

2 teaspoons minced garlic

1 cup bulgur

2½ cups low-sodium chicken stock

½ cup pitted, sliced Kalamata olives

½ cup chopped sun-dried tomatoes

½ cup crumbled feta cheese

¼ cup fresh chopped fresh parsley

1. Preheat the oven to 375°F.

2. Season the chicken thighs with salt and pepper and rub with lemon zest.

3. In a large ovenproof skillet, heat the olive oil over medium-high heat. Sear the chicken until browned, turning once, 8 to 9 minutes. Transfer the chicken to a plate and set aside.

4. In the skillet, combine the onion and garlic and sauté until translucent, about 3 minutes.

5. Stir in the bulgur, chicken stock, olives, and sun-dried tomatoes and bring the mixture to a simmer.

6. Add the chicken thighs back to the skillet, then transfer the skillet, uncovered, to the oven and cook until the bulgur has absorbed all of the stock and the chicken is fully cooked, about 25 minutes. Top with feta cheese and parsley and serve.

SUBSTITUTION TIP: *Swap the bulgur for brown rice or a wild rice blend for a tasty gluten-free meal. Rice is a stellar choice because this dish is a humble one-pot creation that is similar to a pilaf. If you can't find pitted Kalamata olives near you, substitute black olives.*

PER SERVING: *Calories: 402; Total fat: 18g; Saturated fat: 5g; Carbohydrates: 36g; Sugar: 5g; Fiber: 9g; Protein: 28g*

Turkey-Tomato Ragù

SERVES 4 • DAIRY-FREE • MEAL IN ONE

PREP TIME:
10 MINUTES

COOK TIME:
30 MINUTES

Ragù is a classic meat-based Italian sauce usually served with pasta. This version is made with lean ground meat cooked with vegetables and herbs and accented with tomatoes. Celery has a slightly salty taste, so it is often used to reduce added salt in recipes. This elegant vegetable can help detox the body and protect against neurological diseases, heart disease, and cancer.

1 tablespoon olive oil

12 ounces lean ground turkey

3 celery stalks, chopped

1 sweet onion, chopped

1 tablespoon minced garlic

1 (28-ounce) can low-sodium diced tomatoes

1 tablespoon chopped fresh oregano

2 teaspoons chopped fresh basil

8 ounces dry whole-grain linguine

Freshly ground black pepper

1. In a large saucepan, heat the olive oil over medium-high heat. Brown the turkey until cooked through, about 6 minutes.

2. Add the celery, onion, and garlic and sauté until softened, about 4 minutes.

3. Stir in the tomatoes and their juices, oregano, and basil and bring the mixture to a boil. Reduce the heat to low and simmer for 15 minutes.

4. While the sauce is simmering, bring a large pot of water to a boil and cook the pasta according to package instructions until al dente. Drain.

5. Season the sauce with pepper and serve over the pasta.

PER SERVING: *Calories: 432; Total fat: 11g; Saturated fat: 3g; Carbohydrates: 61g; Sugar: 9g; Fiber: 4g; Protein: 27g*

Chickpea-Turkey Stew with Spinach

SERVES 4 • DAIRY-FREE • GLUTEN-FREE • MEAL IN ONE

PREP TIME:
15 MINUTES

COOK TIME:
30 MINUTES

A stew can seem to take forever to cook, so using ground turkey to create one in under an hour is inspired. Cilantro provides much of the bright seasoning in this stew and is used widely in Greek, Spanish, and North African cooking. Cilantro, also known as Chinese parsley, is very rich in vitamins A, B_6, C, and K, manganese, calcium, folate, iron, potassium, and magnesium. If you enjoy this herb, you will benefit with a reduced risk of osteoporosis, diabetes, and heart disease, as well as lowered cholesterol and blood sugar. Cilantro can also help cleanse toxic metals from the body.

1 tablespoon olive oil

1 pound lean ground turkey

1 sweet onion, chopped

2 celery stalks, chopped

2 carrots, peeled and chopped

1 tablespoon minced garlic

2 cups low-sodium chicken stock

2 large tomatoes, chopped

1 (15-ounce) can low-sodium chickpeas, drained and rinsed

1 tablespoon sweet paprika

Dash cayenne pepper

3 cups chopped spinach

Juice of 1 lemon

¼ cup chopped fresh cilantro

Sea salt

Freshly ground black pepper

1. In a large saucepan, heat the olive oil over medium-high heat and brown the ground turkey until cooked through, about 7 minutes.

2. Stir in the onion, celery, carrots, and garlic and sauté for 4 minutes.

Continued >

Chickpea-Turkey Stew with Spinach

Continued

3. Stir in the chicken stock, tomatoes, chickpeas, paprika, and cayenne and bring the stew to a boil. Reduce the heat to low and simmer until the vegetables are tender, about 15 minutes.

4. Stir in the spinach, lemon juice, and cilantro and season with salt and pepper. Let stand for 5 minutes to wilt the spinach and serve.

INGREDIENT TIP: *Substitute diced cooked turkey instead of ground if you have leftover turkey from a holiday dinner. Add about 3 cups to the stew in step 3 along with the chickpeas, and finish the recipe as directed.*

PER SERVING: *Calories: 373; Total fat: 13g; Saturated fat: 3g; Carbohydrates: 36g; Sugar: 3g; Fiber: 8g; Protein: 30g*

Classic Pork Tenderloin Marsala

SERVES 4 • DAIRY-FREE • 30 MINUTES OR LESS

PREP TIME:
10 MINUTES

COOK TIME:
20 MINUTES

Marsala sauce is a rich Italian creation bursting with lightly caramelized mushrooms, garlic, and sweet Marsala wine. You can serve this as is or spoon the sauce over pasta for a more substantial meal. Pork is very high in protein and can be low in fat if you trim the chops before cooking. Pork is high in thiamine, selenium, zinc, B vitamins, phosphorus and iron, a combination that supports a healthy immune system and the cardiovascular system as well as boosts the metabolism.

4 (3-ounce) boneless pork loin chops, trimmed

Sea salt

Freshly ground black pepper

¼ cup whole-wheat flour

1 tablespoon olive oil

2 cups sliced button mushrooms

½ sweet onion, chopped

1 teaspoon minced garlic

½ cup Marsala wine

½ cup low-sodium chicken stock

1 tablespoon cornstarch

1 tablespoon chopped fresh parsley

1. Lightly season the pork chops with salt and pepper.

2. Pour the flour onto a plate and dredge the pork chops to coat both sides, shaking off the excess.

3. In a large skillet, heat the olive oil over medium-high heat and pan-fry the pork chops until cooked through and browned, turning once, about 10 minutes total. Transfer the chops to a plate and set aside.

4. In the skillet, combine the mushrooms, onion, and garlic and sauté until the vegetables are softened, about 5 minutes.

Continued >

5. Stir in the wine, scraping up any bits from the skillet, and bring the liquid to a simmer.

6. In a small bowl, stir together the stock and cornstarch until smooth. Add the stock mixture to the skillet and bring to a boil; cook, stirring, until slightly thickened, about 4 minutes. Serve the chops with the sauce, garnished with parsley.

SUBSTITUTION TIP: *Dredging the pork chops in flour creates a lovely brown crust that can also be achieved with coconut flour or another nut flour, if gluten is a problem. Use any nut or gluten-free flour, or leave this step out completely.*

PER SERVING: *Calories: 200; Total fat: 6g; Saturated fat: 1g; Carbohydrates: 11g; Sugar: 1g; Fiber: 1g; Protein: 20g*

Rosemary-Citrus Roasted Pork Tenderloin

SERVES 4 • DAIRY-FREE • GLUTEN-FREE

PREP TIME:
10 MINUTES, PLUS
MARINATING TIME

COOK TIME:
20 MINUTES

Spanish cuisine often features the main components of this flavorful marinade: rosemary, lemon, and garlic. Rosemary grows wild all over the Mediterranean and has been used to detoxify the liver and improve digestion and blood circulation. This dish can also be made in an oven. Roast the tenderloin on a baking sheet in a 400°F oven until cooked through, 25 to 30 minutes.

¼ cup olive oil

¼ cup chopped fresh rosemary

Juice of 1 lemon

Juice and zest of 1 lime

1 teaspoon minced garlic

1 teaspoon ground cumin

Sea salt

12 ounces boneless pork tenderloin

1. In a medium bowl, whisk together the olive oil, rosemary, lemon juice, lime juice, lime zest, garlic, and cumin. Season with salt. Add the pork tenderloin to the bowl, turning to coat. Cover and refrigerate for 1 hour.

2. Preheat a grill to medium-high heat.

3. Grill the tenderloin, turning several times and basting with the remaining marinade until it is cooked through (internal temperature: 140°F), 15 to 20 minutes.

4. Remove the tenderloin from the grill, cover it with foil, and let rest for 10 minutes. Serve.

PER SERVING: *Calories: 201; Total fat: 15g; Saturated fat: 3g; Carbohydrates: 1g; Sugar: 0g; Fiber: 0g; Protein: 20g*

Chili-Spiced Lamb Chops

SERVES 4 • DAIRY-FREE • GLUTEN-FREE • 30 MINUTES OR LESS

PREP TIME:
2 MINUTES

COOK TIME:
10 MINUTES

Lamb is an extremely common red meat protein in North Africa because beef is not sustainable in that climate and pork is not eaten. The sauce used in this recipe is from Thailand. Chili pastes are found all over the Mediterranean, so you have your choice of flavors and heat levels, but you can use harissa for a more authentic preparation.

4 (4-ounce) loin lamb chops with bones, trimmed

Sea salt

Freshly ground black pepper

1 tablespoon olive oil

2 tablespoons Sriracha sauce

1 tablespoon chopped fresh cilantro

1. Preheat the oven to 450°F.

2. Lightly season the lamb chops with salt and pepper.

3. In a large ovenproof skillet, heat the olive oil over medium-high heat. Brown the chops on both sides, about 2 minutes per side, and spread the chops with sriracha.

4. Place the skillet in the oven and roast until the desired doneness, 4 to 5 minutes for medium. Serve topped with cilantro.

SUBSTITUTION TIP: *This recipe would be equally great if you used pork tenderloin or chicken instead of lamb, in the same amount. You will have to increase the time in the oven to 20 to 25 minutes.*

PER SERVING: *Calories: 223; Total fat: 14g; Saturated fat: 4g; Carbohydrates: 1g; Sugar: 1g; Fiber: 0g; Protein: 23g*

Greek Herbed Beef Meatballs

SERVES 4 • 30 MINUTES OR LESS

PREP TIME:
10 MINUTES

COOK TIME:
20 MINUTES

Meatballs are one of the most versatile dishes because you can use them in a sauce, stuff them into pitas, pile them on a sandwich, and serve them up as a snack with a dip like tzatziki. This beef-based meatball is liberally flavored with lots of fresh herbs, cheese, and garlic. Extra-lean ground beef ensures that the fat content is not too high, but you can also use ground lamb, which is fattier.

1 pound extra-lean ground beef

½ cup panko breadcrumbs

¼ cup grated Parmesan cheese

¼ cup low-fat milk

2 large eggs

1 tablespoon chopped fresh parsley

1 teaspoon chopped fresh oregano

1 teaspoon minced garlic

¼ teaspoon freshly ground black pepper

Sea salt

1. Preheat the oven to 400°F.

2. In a large bowl, combine the ground beef, breadcrumbs, Parmesan cheese, milk, eggs, parsley, oregano, garlic, and pepper. Season lightly with salt.

3. Roll the beef mixture into 1-inch meatballs and arrange on a baking sheet.

4. Bake the meatballs until they are cooked through and browned, turning them several times, about 20 minutes. Serve with a sauce such as Speedy Marinara Sauce (page 191) or stuffed into a pita.

SUBSTITUTION TIP: *Try ground almonds, or any other nut meal, instead of breadcrumbs if gluten is a problem for you or your family. The nuts add a tasty, rich flavor and the texture of the meatballs will not change too much. You might need a bit of water to make the dough stick together.*

PER SERVING: *Calories: 243; Total fat: 8g; Saturated fat: 3g; Carbohydrates: 13g; Sugar: 1g; Fiber: 2g; Protein: 24g*

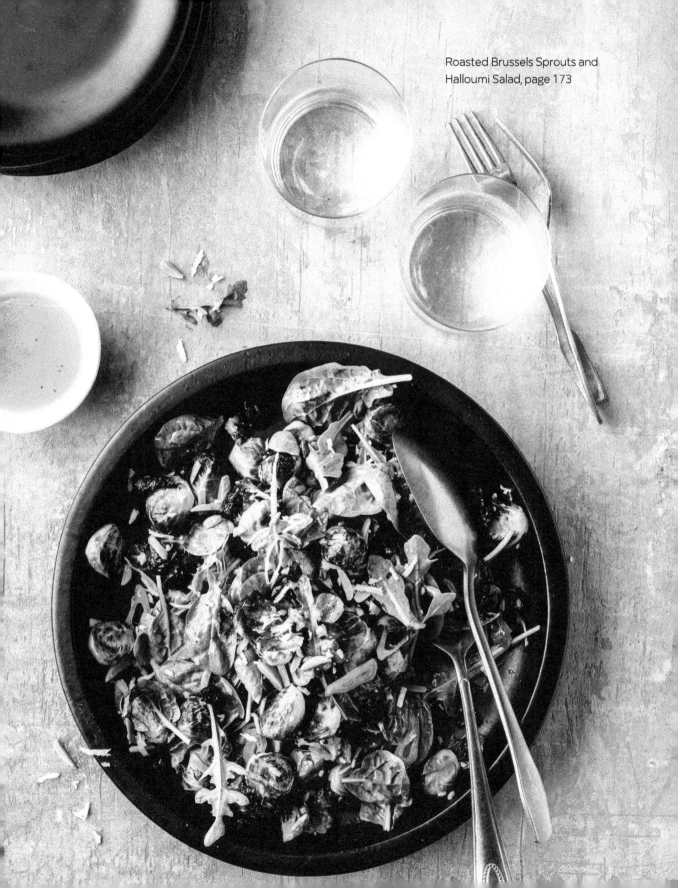

Roasted Brussels Sprouts and
Halloumi Salad, page 173

CHAPTER 11

Vegetables, Grains, and Legumes

Sautéed Dark Leafy Greens 164

Broiled Tomatoes with Feta 165

Parmesan-Sautéed Zucchini with Spaghetti 166

Wild Rice with Grapes 167

Traditional Falafel 168

Spicy Split Pea Tabbouleh 170

Mashed Avocado Egg Salad with Crisps 171

Mediterranean Romaine Wedge Salad 172

Roasted Brussels Sprouts and Halloumi Salad 173

Roasted Vegetable Mélange 175

Couscous-Avocado Salad 176

Sautéed Dark Leafy Greens

SERVES 4 • DAIRY-FREE • GLUTEN-FREE • VEGAN • 30 MINUTES OR LESS

PREP TIME:
10 MINUTES

COOK TIME:
10 MINUTES

Many Mediterranean-inspired dishes feature one type of leafy dark green or another because they are a central component of this healthy lifestyle. Along with the more common greens in this diet, you will often see others, such as dandelion greens, beet greens, watercress, chicory, and purslane. These tender ingredients are packed with nutrients and antioxidants, which support almost every organ and function in the body, as well as reduce the risk of diabetes and most cancers.

2 tablespoons olive oil

8 cups stemmed and coarsely chopped spinach, kale, collard greens, or Swiss chard

Juice of ½ lemon

Sea salt

Freshly ground black pepper

1. In a large skillet, heat the olive oil over medium-high heat. Add the greens and toss with tongs until wilted and tender, 8 to 10 minutes.

2. Remove the skillet from the heat and squeeze in the lemon juice, tossing to coat evenly. Season with salt and pepper and serve.

COOKING TIP: *The volume of chopped greens in your skillet might seem overwhelming at first, but as you toss them, they will soon shrink down and become manageable. If you have a smaller skillet, you can certainly prepare this dish in batches.*

PER SERVING: *Calories: 129; Total fat: 7g; Saturated fat: 1g; Carbohydrates: 14g; Sugar: 0g; Fiber: 2g; Protein: 4g*

Broiled Tomatoes with Feta

SERVES 4 • GLUTEN-FREE • VEGETARIAN • 30 MINUTES OR LESS

PREP TIME:
10 MINUTES

COOK TIME:
8 MINUTES

Tomatoes are used as a vegetable in most recipes, but they are, in fact, a fruit, making them even sweeter when broiled and lightly caramelized with cheese and oil. The addition of basil, a sweet-tasting herb, simply enhances the sublime flavor. Tomatoes are one of those eat-one-a-day ingredients because they provide such a huge amount of the important nutrients for good health. They are a fabulous source of antioxidants, calcium, potassium, vitamins A, B, C, and K, iron, magnesium, malic acid, and oxalic acid. Tomatoes help cleanse the liver, have an anti-aging effect, and reduce the risk of cardiovascular disease, kidney disease, cancer, and hypertension.

4 large tomatoes, cut in half horizontally

1 tablespoon olive oil

1 teaspoon minced garlic

½ cup crumbled feta cheese

1 tablespoon chopped fresh basil

Sea salt

Freshly ground black pepper

1. Preheat the oven to broil.

2. Place the tomato halves, cut-side up, in a 9-by-13-inch baking dish and drizzle them with the olive oil. Rub the garlic into the tomatoes.

3. Broil the tomatoes for about 5 minutes, until softened. Sprinkle with the feta cheese and broil for 3 minutes longer.

4. Sprinkle with basil and season with salt and pepper. Serve.

COOKING TIP: *If you are using the grill for the main part of your meal, grill the tomatoes instead of broiling them. Oil the grill, place the tomatoes cut-side down, and grill for 4 to 5 minutes, until lightly charred and softened. Turn them over and top with the feta cheese. Remove from the heat and serve.*

PER SERVING: *Calories: 113; Total fat: 8g; Saturated fat: 3g; Carbohydrates: 8g; Sugar: 6g; Fiber: 2g; Protein: 4g*

Parmesan-Sautéed Zucchini with Spaghetti

SERVES 4 • VEGETARIAN • 30 MINUTES OR LESS • MEAL IN ONE

PREP TIME:
10 MINUTES

COOK TIME:
15 MINUTES

Humble zucchini becomes something exceptional when sautéed with nutty, tangy Parmesan cheese and garlic. The hearty pasta tossed with tender vegetables, browned cheese bits, and aromatic garlic needs no other accompaniments. Zucchini, both green and yellow, reduces the risk of cancer, stroke, kidney disease, arthritis, diabetes, and gout. The best zucchini are dark green in color, slightly glossy, and free of blemishes and wrinkles. They should also feel slightly heavy for their size.

8 ounces dry whole-grain spaghetti

2 tablespoons olive oil

1 tablespoon minced garlic

4 zucchini, chopped

½ cup grated Parmesan cheese, divided

Sea salt

Freshly ground black pepper

1. Bring a large pot of water to a boil and cook the pasta according to the package instructions until al dente. Drain.

2. While the pasta is cooking, in a large skillet, heat the olive oil over medium-high heat. Sauté the garlic until softened, about 2 minutes.

3. Add the zucchini and sauté until the squash is lightly caramelized, about 5 minutes. Stir in ¼ cup of Parmesan cheese and toss until the cheese is melted and lightly browned.

4. Add the cooked spaghetti to the skillet and toss to coat. Season with salt and pepper and serve topped with the remaining ¼ cup of Parmesan cheese.

PER SERVING: *Calories: 338; Total fat: 11g; Saturated fat: 3g; Carbohydrates: 50g; Sugar: 3g; Fiber: 2g; Protein: 15g*

Wild Rice with Grapes

SERVES 4 • DAIRY-FREE • GLUTEN-FREE • VEGAN

PREP TIME:
10 MINUTES

COOK TIME:
50 MINUTES

This dish has texture, a tart-sweet taste, and a hint of floral thyme. The wild rice mix can be replaced with straight wild rice or just brown rice. Grapes might seem like an odd choice for a side dish, but their sweetness is lovely combined with nutty, earthy wild rice. Grapes are very high in antioxidants, including resveratrol, as well as folate, beta-carotene, manganese, iron, and vitamins A, B_1, B_2, B_6, C, E, and K. Red grapes can reduce the risk of blood clots and lower cholesterol and blood pressure.

1 cup wild rice blend

1¾ cups water

1 teaspoon olive oil

2 cups red seedless grapes

2 teaspoons chopped fresh thyme

Sea salt

Freshly ground black pepper

1. In a pot, combine the rice and water and bring to a boil. Cover, reduce the heat to low, and simmer for 45 minutes. Remove from the heat and let stand, covered, for 10 minutes. Fluff with a fork.

2. In a large skillet, heat the olive oil over medium-high heat.

3. Add the grapes and thyme and sauté until the grapes begin to burst, about 5 minutes.

4. Stir in the wild rice mixture and season with salt and pepper. Serve.

INGREDIENT TIP: *Wild rice is not rice at all; it is the seed of a water grass that is indigenous to North America. You can find both cultivated and authentic handpicked wild rice in your local store. Cultivated wild rice is less expensive and has a milder taste and dark ebony color. It will work fine in this recipe and is usually the type found in premixed rice blends.*

PER SERVING: *Calories: 146; Total fat: 2g; Saturated fat: 0g; Carbohydrates: 31g; Sugar: 12g; Fiber: 2g; Protein: 3g*

Traditional Falafel

SERVES 4 • DAIRY-FREE • MEAL IN ONE • VEGAN • 30 MINUTES OR LESS

PREP TIME:
20 MINUTES

COOK TIME:
10 MINUTES

Falafel is a traditional chickpea or fava bean dish with an origin that has been hotly contested by Israel, Egypt, Lebanon, and several other Middle Eastern countries. Regardless of where this tasty golden creation originated, it is a staple in many Mediterranean countries. This version uses chickpeas with heaps of parsley and cilantro and a dash of citrus and nutty cumin. Chickpeas are extremely high in soluble fiber, resistant starch, and protein, so they can increase feelings of satiety. Eating chickpeas creates an improved glycemic response and stimulates the body to release an appetite-suppressing hormone called cholecystokinin.

1 (15-ounce) can low-sodium chickpeas, drained and rinsed

½ sweet onion, chopped

¼ cup whole-wheat flour

¼ cup coarsely chopped fresh parsley

¼ cup coarsely chopped fresh cilantro

Juice from 1 lemon

1 tablespoon minced garlic

2 teaspoon ground cumin

Sea salt

Freshly ground black pepper

2 tablespoons olive oil

1. In a food processor, pulse the chickpeas, onion, flour, parsley, cilantro, lemon juice, garlic, and cumin until the mixture just holds together. Season with salt and pepper and mix again.

2. Scoop out about 2 tablespoons of the mixture, roll into a ball, and flatten it out slightly to form a thick patty. Repeat with the remaining chickpea mixture.

3. In a large skillet, heat the olive oil over medium-high heat and pan-fry the patties until golden brown, about 4 minutes per side. Serve alone or stuffed into pita bread.

COOKING TIP: *Falafel can be made ahead and either frozen before cooking or frozen after browning. Place the patties on a baking sheet and freeze them completely before transferring them to sealable plastic freezer bags. Take out the amount you want to use and defrost in the refrigerator overnight.*

PER SERVING: *Calories: 245; Total fat: 9g; Saturated fat: 1g; Carbohydrates: 36g; Sugar: 1g; Fiber: 6g; Protein: 7g*

Spicy Split Pea Tabbouleh

SERVES 6 • DAIRY-FREE • GLUTEN-FREE • MEAL IN ONE • VEGAN

PREP TIME:
15 MINUTES,
PLUS 1 HOUR
CHILLING TIME

COOK TIME:
45 MINUTES

Split peas are generally not available precooked in convenient cans. But they are highly nutritious, and this tasty tabbouleh is completely worth the effort of cooking them.

1½ cups split peas

4 cups water

2 large tomatoes, seeded and chopped

1 English cucumber, chopped

1 yellow bell pepper, chopped

1 orange bell pepper, chopped

½ red onion, finely chopped

¼ cup chopped fresh cilantro

Juice of 1 lime

1 teaspoon ground cumin

½ teaspoon ground coriander

Pinch red pepper flakes

Sea salt

Freshly ground black pepper

1. In a large saucepan, combine the split peas and water over medium-high heat and bring to a boil. Reduce the heat to low and simmer, uncovered, until the peas are tender, 40 to 45 minutes. Drain the peas and rinse them in cold water to cool.

2. Transfer the peas to a large bowl and add the tomatoes, cucumber, bell peppers, onion, cilantro, lime juice, cumin, coriander, and red pepper flakes. Toss to mix well. Place the mixture in the refrigerator for at least 1 hour to let the flavors mesh. Season with salt and pepper and serve.

PER SERVING: *Calories: 208; Total fat: 1g; Saturated fat: 0g; Carbohydrates: 38g; Sugar: 7g; Fiber: 14g; Protein: 14g*

Mashed Avocado Egg Salad with Crisps

SERVES 4 • DAIRY-FREE • MEAL IN ONE • VEGETARIAN • 30 MINUTES OR LESS

PREP TIME:
20 MINUTES

Avocado and egg make for a striking and appetizing combination. Add scarlet tomatoes and dark green parsley, and you have a masterpiece. The protein and healthy fats will fill you up and provide energy all day. Try pita bread, grilled tortillas, or even large lettuce leaves as the base for this dish instead of toast.

6 hard-boiled eggs, peeled and coarsely chopped

1 avocado, peeled and pitted

1 celery stalk, chopped

Juice and zest of ½ lemon

1 teaspoon chopped fresh parsley

4 whole-wheat bread slices, toasted

2 tomatoes, thinly sliced

Sea salt

Freshly ground black pepper

1. In a medium bowl, mash the eggs and avocado until well blended but still chunky. Stir in the celery, lemon juice, lemon zest, and parsley until well mixed.

2. Generously spread the egg mixture on the toast and arrange the tomato slices on top. Season with salt and pepper and serve.

COOKING TIP: *Make the hard-boiled eggs ahead of time and store in the refrigerator for up to 1 week. Use eggs that are at least 7 days old because they are more alkaline and will peel easier, or add 1 teaspoon of baking soda to the water when boiling if your eggs are fresher.*

PER SERVING: *Calories: 248; Total fat: 14g; Saturated fat: 3g; Carbohydrates: 18g; Sugar: 4g; Fiber: 6g; Protein: 13g*

Mediterranean Romaine Wedge Salad

SERVES 4 • GLUTEN-FREE • MEAL IN ONE • VEGETARIAN • 30 MINUTES OR LESS

PREP TIME:
25 MINUTES

Wedge salads look absolutely beautiful on the plate. Fennel is popular in French, Spanish, Italian, and Greek cooking. Fennel has a licorice-like taste that can take a bit of time to get used to, but it is packed with vitamin C, potassium, iron, and B vitamins and is high in manganese, magnesium, vitamin E, and copper. This root vegetable can reduce symptoms associated with menopause, support a healthy digestive system, and combat depression.

1 English cucumber, chopped

1 cup quartered cherry tomatoes

1 cup chopped fennel

½ cup chopped roasted red peppers

¼ cup pitted, halved Kalamata olives

1 scallion, both white and green parts, chopped

½ cup Pesto Vinaigrette (page 190), divided

2 romaine lettuce heads, cut in half lengthwise

¼ cup grated Asiago cheese

2 tablespoons chopped fresh basil

1. In a large bowl, stir together the cucumber, tomatoes, fennel, roasted red peppers, olives, scallion, and ¼ cup of pesto vinaigrette.

2. Place each romaine half on a large plate. Evenly divide the vegetable mixture onto each wedge.

3. Drizzle the remaining dressing over the romaine wedges.

4. Serve topped with Asiago cheese and basil.

SUBSTITUTION TIP: *Leave out the Asiago cheese for a dairy-free recipe and instead use grated hard-boiled eggs as a topping.*

PER SERVING: *Calories: 336; Total fat: 27g; Saturated fat: 5g; Carbohydrates: 23g; Sugar: 7g; Fiber: 2g; Protein: 11g*

Roasted Brussels Sprouts and Halloumi Salad

SERVES 4 • GLUTEN-FREE • MEAL IN ONE • VEGETARIAN

PREP TIME:
10 MINUTES

COOK TIME:
35 MINUTES

Halloumi is a sheep's milk cheese hailing from the Greek island of Cyprus. The soft, curd-like cheese is made without using rennet, so it is a great choice for vegetarians who wish to avoid rennet. Brussels sprouts are loaded with fiber, vitamin K, and vitamin C.

FOR THE DRESSING

¼ cup olive oil

⅓ cup freshly squeezed lemon juice

2 tablespoons honey

1 teaspoon mustard

Sea salt

Freshly ground black pepper

FOR THE SALAD

2 pounds Brussels sprouts, trimmed and halved

2 tablespoons olive oil

1 teaspoon sea salt

1½ cups baby spinach

½ cup baby arugula

1 shallot, halved and thinly sliced

3 tablespoons dried cranberries

½ cup blanched almonds, toasted

¼ cup shredded halloumi cheese

TO MAKE THE DRESSING

In a small bowl, whisk together the olive oil, lemon juice, honey, and mustard. Season with salt and pepper and set aside.

Continued >

Roasted Brussels Sprouts and Halloumi Salad

Continued

1. Preheat the oven to 425°F.

2. Put the Brussels sprouts in a large mixing bowl. Drizzle with olive oil and season with salt. Toss to combine. Spread the Brussels sprouts on a large baking sheet. Roast for 25 to 30 minutes, stirring once about halfway through, until crispy on the outside and tender on the inside.

3. While the Brussels sprouts are roasting, in a large mixing bowl, combine the spinach, arugula, shallot, cranberries, and almonds. Once cooked, add the roasted Brussels sprouts to the bowl.

4. Pour the dressing on the salad and toss to combine. Add shredded halloumi cheese and give it another gentle toss. Transfer the salad to a large serving platter.

SUBSTITUTION TIP: *If you are unable to get your hands on halloumi cheese, crumbled goat cheese is a good alternative.*

PER SERVING: *Calories: 475; Total fat: 34g; Saturated fat: 6g; Carbohydrates: 41g; Sugar: 20g; Fiber: 12g; Protein: 14g*

Roasted Vegetable Mélange

SERVES 4 • DAIRY-FREE • GLUTEN-FREE • MEAL IN ONE • VEGAN

PREP TIME:
20 MINUTES

COOK TIME:
25 MINUTES

Assorted roasted vegetables can be a filling main meal or side dish, depending on your needs and the amount you prepare. All the essential nutrient groups are covered with the produce in this recipe, including every vitamin and mineral, fiber, protein, and a plethora of powerful antioxidants and phytonutrients.

½ cauliflower head, cut into small florets

½ broccoli head, cut into small florets

2 zucchini, cut into ½-inch pieces

2 cups halved mushrooms

2 red, orange, or yellow bell peppers, cut into 1-inch pieces

1 sweet potato, cut into 1-inch pieces

1 red onion, cut into wedges

3 tablespoons olive oil

2 teaspoons minced garlic

1 teaspoon chopped fresh thyme

Sea salt

Freshly ground black pepper

1. Preheat the oven to 400°F. Line a baking sheet with parchment paper and set aside.

2. In a large bowl, toss the cauliflower, broccoli, zucchini, mushrooms, bell peppers, sweet potato, onion, olive oil, garlic, and thyme until well mixed. Spread the vegetables on the baking sheet and season lightly with salt and pepper.

3. Roast until the vegetables are tender and lightly caramelized, stirring occasionally, 20 to 25 minutes. Serve.

PER SERVING: *Calories: 183; Total fat: 11g; Saturated fat: 2g; Carbohydrates: 20g; Sugar: 8g; Fiber: 6g; Protein: 5g*

Couscous-Avocado Salad

SERVES 4 • MEAL IN ONE • VEGETARIAN

PREP TIME:
15 MINUTES,
PLUS 1 HOUR
CHILLING TIME

COOK TIME:
10 MINUTES

Avocado is not a native Mediterranean fruit, but it fits very well into this diet plan with its monounsaturated fat, fiber, omega-3 fatty acids, beta-carotene, lutein, vitamins, and minerals. Combining avocado with cherry tomatoes can increase the absorption of lycopene from the tomatoes by 300 to 400 percent because lycopene is fat-soluble. Avocado promotes liver health, reduces inflammation in the body, and lowers the risk of cancer and heart disease.

FOR THE DRESSING

¼ cup olive oil

2 tablespoons red wine vinegar

1 teaspoon minced garlic

1 teaspoon chopped fresh oregano

Pinch red pepper flakes

Sea salt

Freshly ground black pepper

FOR THE SALAD

1 cup couscous

2 cups halved cherry tomatoes

½ English cucumber, chopped

1 cup chopped marinated artichoke hearts

1 avocado, pitted, peeled, and chopped

½ cup crumbled feta cheese

2 tablespoons pine nuts

In a small bowl, whisk together the olive oil, vinegar, garlic, oregano, and red pepper flakes. Season with salt and pepper and set aside.

1. In a pot, bring 1½ cups of water to a boil. Stir the couscous into the boiling water and remove from the heat. Cover and let sit for 10 minutes. Fluff with a fork.

2. In a large bowl, toss together the couscous, cherry tomatoes, cucumber, artichoke hearts, avocado, feta cheese, and pine nuts. Add the dressing and toss to combine. Refrigerate for 1 hour and serve.

COOKING TIP: *There are many types of couscous available in the store, but the best for this salad is the larger pea-size Israeli or pearl couscous. Simmer 1 cup of Israeli couscous with 1¼ cups of water or broth for about 10 minutes, covered, and then fluff with a fork.*

PER SERVING: *Calories: 489; Total fat: 30g; Saturated fat: 6g; Carbohydrates: 46g; Sugar: 4g; Fiber: 7g; Protein: 11g*

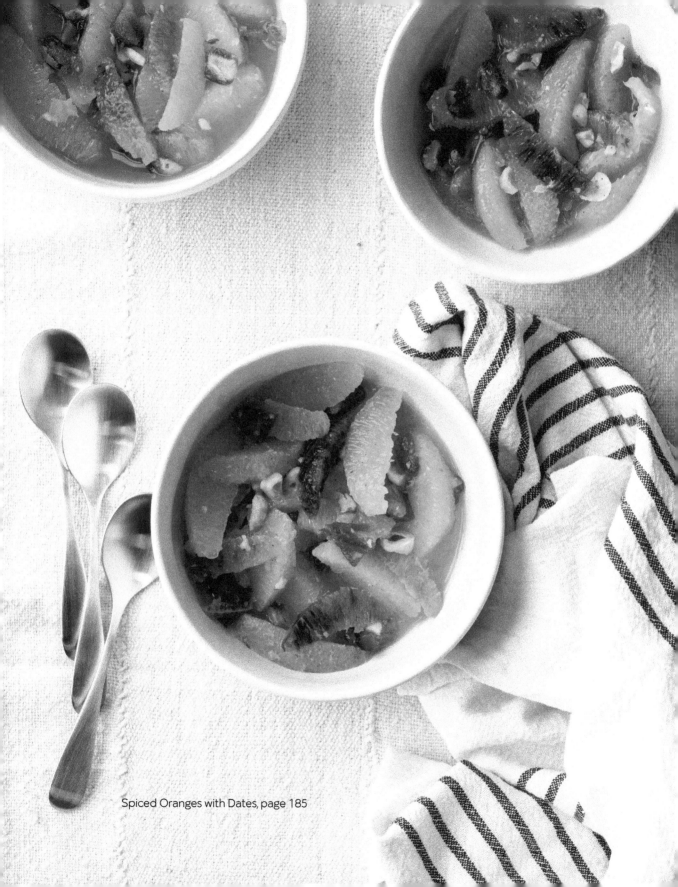

Spiced Oranges with Dates, page 185

CHAPTER 12

Snacks and Sweets

Balsamic Vinegar-Marinated Strawberries 180

Fruit-Topped Meringues 181

Light Greek Yogurt Chocolate Pudding 182

Pomegranate Granita 183

Creamy Panna Cotta 184

Spiced Oranges with Dates 185

Balsamic Vinegar-Marinated Strawberries

SERVES 4 • DAIRY-FREE • GLUTEN-FREE • VEGETARIAN • 30 MINUTES OR LESS

PREP TIME:
15 MINUTES,
PLUS 15 MINUTES
CHILLING TIME

Ripe strawberries and tart balsamic vinegar probably seem like an unlikely pairing, but this combination creates an incredible flavor burst in your mouth. Strawberries are one of the most popular fruits in the world for a good reason—they are delicious and nutritious. Strawberries are very high in ellagic acid, beta-carotene, potassium, and vitamins A and C. Eating this pretty berry can boost your immune system and help stabilize your blood sugar, as well as reduce the risk of many cancers, heart disease, and cognitive decline.

⅓ cup balsamic vinegar

1 tablespoon honey

2 teaspoons pure vanilla extract

8 cups hulled and halved strawberries

1. In a medium bowl, whisk together the balsamic vinegar, honey, and vanilla until blended. Stir in the strawberries and let the berries marinate in the refrigerator for 15 minutes.

2. Drain the vinegar mixture out of the strawberries and serve immediately.

INGREDIENT TIP: *Look for strawberries that are a deep red color with no pale green or yellow areas on them. Strawberries do not ripen after they're picked, so these discolorations mean they are immature and most likely sour. Buy your berries the day before or on the day you need them because they are extremely perishable.*

PER SERVING: *Calories: 138; Total fat: 1g; Saturated fat: 0g; Carbohydrates: 32g; Sugar: 22g; Fiber: 6g; Protein: 2g*

Fruit-Topped Meringues

MAKES 24 COOKIES • DAIRY-FREE • GLUTEN-FREE • VEGETARIAN

PREP TIME:
15 MINUTES,
PLUS 1 HOUR
COOLING TIME

COOK TIME:
50 MINUTES

Meringues' crunchy exterior and delicately sweet melt-in-the-mouth interior make a perfect base for raspberries, which are high in manganese and vitamins B, C, E, and K and are a good source of beta-carotene, calcium, potassium, and ellagic acid. They can promote healthy skin and reduce the risk of heart disease, liver fibrosis, Parkinson's disease, and cancer.

4 large egg whites, at room temperature

¼ teaspoon cream of tartar

Pinch sea salt

½ cup honey

1 cup raspberries

1. Preheat the oven to 200°F. Line two baking sheets with parchment paper and set aside.

2. In a large stainless steel bowl, beat the egg whites until they are frothy.

3. Beat in the cream of tartar and salt until soft peaks form, 4 to 5 minutes.

4. Beat in the honey, 1 tablespoon at a time, until stiff glossy peaks form.

5. Spoon the meringue batter onto the baking sheets by tablespoons and create a small well in the center of each with the back of a spoon.

6. Bake until firm, 45 to 50 minutes. Turn off the heat in the oven and prop the door open to cool the meringues in the oven for at least 1 hour.

7. Store in an airtight container for up to 1 week and serve with a raspberry in the center of each meringue.

COOKING TIP: *For a special presentation, spoon the meringue batter into a piping bag fitted with an open star tip and pipe the meringue cookies instead of using a spoon. You can pipe the batter into the shape of a disc with a ring around it so there is a space on the disc for the fruit topping.*

PER SERVING (2 COOKIES): *Calories: 54; Total fat: 0g; Saturated fat: 0g; Carbohydrates: 13g; Sugar: 12g; Fiber: 1g; Protein: 1g*

Light Greek Yogurt Chocolate Pudding

SERVES 4 • GLUTEN-FREE • VEGETARIAN

PREP TIME:
10 MINUTES,
PLUS 3 HOURS
CHILLING TIME

COOK TIME:
5 MINUTES

C hocolate is an obsession for many, a pleasure that is thankfully healthy for you in small amounts. Chocolate has many of the benefits of dark leafy vegetables, such as antioxidants and flavonoids, which are extremely beneficial for the heart. Dark chocolate has been proven to lower cholesterol and blood pressure by impressive amounts. Consuming cocoa can improve nitric acid activity, which in turn helps maintain blood pressure. The flavonols in the cocoa can also stop platelets from clotting together, which is similar to the effect of taking an aspirin.

½ cup unsweetened almond milk

4 ounces dark chocolate, at least 60 percent cacao, coarsely chopped

2 cups low-fat plain Greek yogurt

1 teaspoon pure vanilla extract

Whipped coconut cream, for garnish

1. In a saucepan, bring about 1-inch of water to a simmer over low heat. Place a small heat-resistant bowl over the saucepan.

2. Add the almond milk and chocolate to the bowl and stir until the chocolate is completely melted and the mixture is smooth, about 5 minutes.

3. Remove the bowl from the heat and whisk in the yogurt and vanilla until well blended. Cover the pudding with plastic wrap and chill in the refrigerator for at least 3 hours. Serve topped with whipped coconut cream.

SUBSTITUTION TIP: *Coconut and soy yogurts have come a long way in flavor and texture and can be used in place of "real" yogurt in most recipes to create a vegan dessert. Make sure you read the ingredient label on the yogurt to make sure gelatin is not a thickener.*

PER SERVING: *Calories: 238; Total fat: 11g; Saturated fat: 6g; Carbohydrates: 21g; Sugar: 17g; Fiber: 2g; Protein: 13g*

Pomegranate Granita

SERVES 4 • DAIRY-FREE • GLUTEN-FREE • VEGETARIAN

PREP TIME:
6 MINUTES,
PLUS 4 HOURS
CHILLING TIME

Granita is a frozen dessert related to sorbet and Italian ice that originated in Sicily and is characterized by a coarse, large ice crystal texture. It is made from fruit, water, sweeteners, and flavorings, like the ground cinnamon in this recipe. Cinnamon is a sweet, fragrant spice that cuts the tartness of the pomegranate perfectly. Cinnamon has a long history of healing with the essential oils of its bark, cinnamaldehyde, cinnamyl acetate, and cinnamyl alcohol, along with vitamin K, iron, manganese, and calcium. This spice can help normalize blood sugar, improve brain activity, lower the risk of heart disease and cholesterol, and support a healthy digestive system.

4 cups pure pomegranate juice (no sugar added)

¼ cup honey

¼ teaspoon ground cinnamon

Pinch sea salt

1. In a medium bowl, whisk together the pomegranate juice, honey, cinnamon, and salt until well blended. Pour the pomegranate mixture into a 9-by-13-by-3-inch metal baking dish.

2. Freeze the mixture for at least 4 hours, scraping the surface with a fork every 30 minutes or so until the mixture looks like colored snow. Store the granita in the freezer in a sealed container for up to 2 weeks, scraping with a fork when you want to serve it.

SUBSTITUTION TIP: *You can make granita with almost any type of juice or puréed fruit, so let your imagination run wild. Blood orange juice, watermelon, and ruby red grapefruit juice all create lovely vibrant mixtures. Adjust the honey to suit the sweetness of whatever fruit you try in this recipe.*

PER SERVING: *Calories: 205; Total fat: 0g; Saturated fat: 0g; Carbohydrates: 56g; Sugar: 54g; Fiber: 0g; Protein: 0g*

Creamy Panna Cotta

SERVES 4 • GLUTEN-FREE

PREP TIME:
10 MINUTES,
PLUS 3 HOURS
CHILLING TIME

COOK TIME:
2 MINUTES

Panna cotta, or "cooked cream," is a classic Italian dessert. This version is sweetened with honey, which has nutrients and vitamins missing in refined sugars. Honey is a natural energy booster and can combat muscle fatigue due to exertion. Honey contains many powerful antioxidants and antibacterial properties, which are very beneficial for the immune system. It can positively impact a broad variety of ailments from arthritis to cardiovascular disease.

½ cup unsweetened almond milk

1 (¼-ounce) packet unflavored gelatin

1½ cups low-fat milk

¼ cup honey

1 teaspoon cornstarch

½ teaspoon almond extract

1 cup fresh berries

1. Pour the almond milk into a small saucepan and sprinkle the gelatin over it; let stand for 5 minutes.

2. Place the saucepan over medium-low heat and heat until the gelatin is dissolved, about 2 minutes. Remove from the heat and whisk in the milk, honey, cornstarch, and almond extract.

3. Pour the panna cotta mixture into 4 (6-ounce) ramekins and wrap them in plastic wrap. Refrigerate until set, about 3 hours.

4. Loosen the panna cotta by running a knife around the inside edges of the ramekins and invert them onto serving plates. Top with berries and serve.

INGREDIENT TIP: *Honey's flavor changes depending on the type of flowers bees have access to when collecting nectar, so the type you choose can significantly impact the taste of this dessert. If looking for a stronger, full-bodied taste, try buckwheat honey; for a delicate, almost flowery flavor, use alfalfa honey.*

PER SERVING: *Calories: 129; Total fat: 1g; Saturated fat: 1g; Carbohydrates: 26g; Sugar: 24g; Fiber: 1g; Protein: 5g*

Spiced Oranges with Dates

SERVES 4 • DAIRY-FREE • GLUTEN-FREE • VEGAN • 30 MINUTES OR LESS

PREP TIME:
15 MINUTES

Desserts don't have to be elaborate creations full of sugar and saturated fats; the end of your meal can be light and simple. One orange contains the minimum recommended daily amount of vitamin C for an adult and is also a wonderful source of vitamin A, limonoid, iron, and calcium. Citrus can help boost your immune system, combat the common cold, and lower cholesterol.

4 large oranges

2 large blood oranges or cara cara oranges

¼ cup coarsely chopped Medjool dates

⅛ teaspoon ground cloves

2 tablespoons chopped hazelnuts

1. Use a sharp paring knife to cut the skin and pith off the oranges so you just have the flesh. Follow the membranes to cut the sections of the oranges out, and place in a medium bowl. Squeeze any remaining juice from the membranes into the bowl with the fruit.

2. Add the dates, cloves, and hazelnuts to the bowl and toss to combine.

3. Store in a sealed container in the refrigerator. Serve spooned into individual bowls.

INGREDIENT TIP: *Blood oranges are usually in season from early winter to spring, so that is the time they will be most affordable. Look for oranges that feel firm and heavy for their size because that indicates the fruit is juicy. Ripe blood oranges can have a little green tint to the rind, but this will not affect their taste.*

PER SERVING: *Calories: 184; Total fat: 2g; Saturated fat: 0g; Carbohydrates: 43g; Sugar: 35g; Fiber: 8g; Protein: 3g*

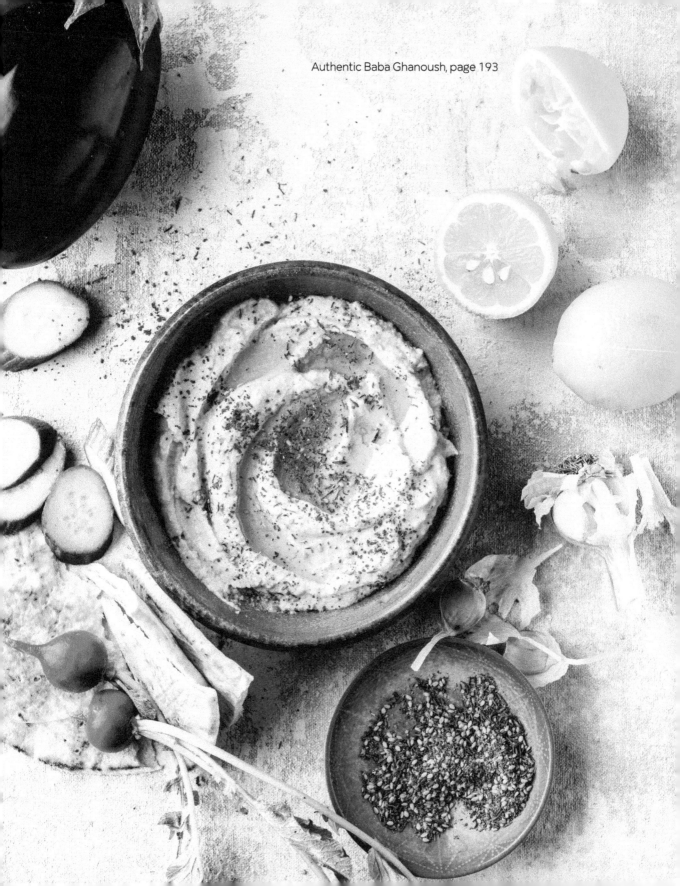

Authentic Baba Ghanoush, page 193

CHAPTER 13

Dressings and Dips

Traditional Hummus   188

Roasted Garlic   189

Pesto Vinaigrette   190

Speedy Marinara Sauce   191

Tzatziki Sauce   192

Authentic Baba Ghanoush   193

Traditional Hummus

MAKES 3 CUPS • DAIRY-FREE • GLUTEN-FREE • VEGAN • 30 MINUTES OR LESS

PREP TIME:
10 MINUTES

Hummus is the Arabic word for chickpea, but this popular ancient dip can be made with other types of beans as well as vegetables such as kale, sweet potato, pumpkin, or cauliflower. This garlic- and tahini-laced chickpea dip is perfect for any event and as a tasty spread for wraps and sandwiches.

2 (15-ounce) cans low-sodium chickpeas, drained and rinsed

3 garlic cloves, peeled

¼ cup tahini

½ cup olive oil

Juice of 1 lemon

¼ teaspoon sea salt

1. In a food processor, combine the chickpeas, garlic, tahini, olive oil, lemon juice, and salt and pulse until chopped. Scrape down the sides and purée until the mixture is smooth.

2. Serve with pita bread or crudités. Store for up to 1 week in a sealed container in the refrigerator.

INGREDIENT TIP: *If you have any leftover chickpeas, store them in the refrigerator in a sealed container for up to a week. Use the chickpeas in salads and stews or try roasting your extras in the oven for a crispy nutritious snack.*

PER SERVING (¼ CUP): *Calories: 170; Total fat: 12g; Saturated fat: 2g; Carbohydrates: 13g; Sugar: 2g; Fiber: 4g; Protein: 5g*

Roasted Garlic

MAKES 1 CUP • GLUTEN-FREE • VEGETARIAN • 30 MINUTES OR LESS

PREP TIME:
2 MINUTES

COOK TIME:
25 MINUTES

Roasted garlic is so utterly delectable it is often served in Mediterranean countries spread liberally on crusty bread as an appetizer. The health benefits of garlic are relatively well known, and this pungent allium has been used for centuries to heal the body. Garlic contains 12 antioxidants, amino acids, allicin, iron, potassium, and vitamins A, B$_6$, and C, and is rich in calcium, selenium, and manganese. As a superfood, garlic helps detoxify the body and supports a healthy cardiovascular system by lowering cholesterol, blood pressure, and the risk of blood clots.

2 cups peeled garlic cloves

½ cup low-fat milk

1 tablespoon olive oil

1. Preheat the oven to 350°F.

2. In a medium ovenproof skillet, combine the garlic and milk and bring to a boil over medium-high heat. Reduce the heat to low and simmer for 5 minutes, stirring occasionally.

3. Remove the skillet from the heat, drain the milk, and stir in the olive oil. Cover the skillet with foil and roast garlic in the oven until very tender and golden, about 20 minutes. Store roasted garlic in a sealed container in the refrigerator for up to 1 week.

SUBSTITUTION TIP: *If you need a vegan-friendly roasted garlic, do not blanch the cloves in milk because this step is not crucial. The milk adds a certain lush sweetness to the roasted garlic and leeches out any sharpness of flavor if your cloves are a bit green.*

PER SERVING (1 TABLESPOON): *Calories: 37; Total fat: 1g; Saturated fat: 0g; Carbohydrates: 6g; Sugar: 0g; Fiber: 0g; Protein: 1g*

Pesto Vinaigrette

MAKES ¾ CUP • DAIRY-FREE • GLUTEN-FREE • VEGAN • 30 MINUTES OR LESS

PREP TIME:
10 MINUTES

This all-purpose vinaigrette can be used as a dressing for salads and side dishes, a dip for cut-up veggies, and a marinade for fish, poultry, and meats. The apple cider vinegar has many health benefits, so you will be getting more than just a delicious vinaigrette. Apple cider vinegar can help promote proper digestion because it can permeate the intestinal tract and eliminate the harmful bacteria that disrupt digestion.

¼ cup apple cider vinegar

2 tablespoons basil pesto

½ cup olive oil

Sea salt

Freshly ground black pepper

In a medium bowl, whisk the vinegar and pesto together until blended. Add the olive oil in a thin stream while whisking until the vinaigrette is emulsified and season with salt and pepper. Store dressing in a sealed container in the refrigerator for up to 1 week.

SUBSTITUTION TIP: *Any type of pesto is fabulous in this vinaigrette, so feel free to use whatever you have in the refrigerator. Use sun-dried tomato pesto, artichoke pesto, cilantro pesto, or kale pesto in the same amount to create different variations. Experiment to discover your favorite.*

PER SERVING (2 TABLESPOONS): *Calories: 175; Total fat: 20g; Saturated fat: 3g; Carbohydrates: 2g; Sugar: 0g; Fiber: 0g; Protein: 1g*

Speedy Marinara Sauce

MAKES 4 CUPS • DAIRY-FREE • GLUTEN-FREE • VEGAN

PREP TIME:
10 MINUTES

COOK TIME:
25 MINUTES

This marinara sauce is garlicky, rich, and packed with fresh herb flavor. Tomatoes owe their gorgeous red color to an antioxidant called lycopene, which can reduce the risk of several types of cancer, such as bladder, breast, lung, and prostate, as well as prevent heart disease. This antioxidant is hard for the body to digest when tomatoes are raw, so cooking them in olive oil along with the other sauce ingredients can increase the absorption of the lycopene.

1 tablespoon olive oil

1 sweet onion, finely chopped

1 tablespoon minced garlic

2 (15-ounce) cans low-sodium crushed tomatoes

2 tablespoons chopped fresh basil

2 tablespoons chopped fresh oregano

Sea salt

Freshly ground black pepper

1. In a large saucepan, heat the olive oil over medium-high heat. Sauté the onion and garlic until softened and lightly caramelized, about 5 minutes.

2. Stir in the tomatoes and their juices and bring the mixture to a gentle boil. Reduce the heat to low and simmer, covered, for 15 to 20 minutes.

3. Remove the saucepan from the heat and stir in the basil and oregano. Season with salt and pepper. Serve immediately or chill and store in the refrigerator in a sealed container for up to 1 week.

INGREDIENT TIP: *Basil often comes in large bunches, so you will probably have some left over. Wash and chop the basil and divide among ice cube tray sections. Cover the herbs with water and freeze until firm. Pop the cubes out and transfer them to a freezer bag. When ready to use, add the entire ice cube to soups, sauces, and stews.*

PER SERVING: *Calories: 91; Total fat: 4g; Saturated fat: 1g; Carbohydrates: 13g; Sugar: 5g; Fiber: 3g; Protein: 2g*

Tzatziki Sauce

MAKES 2 CUPS • GLUTEN-FREE • VEGETARIAN • 30 MINUTES OR LESS

PREP TIME:
10 MINUTES

The word "refreshing" does not do this pretty pale green dip justice. Cool cucumber, citrus, and tangy yogurt create a glorious taste sensation you might want to finish off with a spoon. Cucumber is a popular detox ingredient because it is a powerful diuretic that can help reduce the signs of aging and inflammation in the body. Cucumbers are also an excellent source of vitamins A and C, calcium, and beta-carotene.

1 cup low-fat plain Greek yogurt

1 large English cucumber, grated, with all the liquid squeezed out

3 tablespoons chopped fresh dill

2 tablespoons freshly squeezed lemon juice

1 teaspoon minced garlic

Sea salt

Freshly ground black pepper

In a medium bowl, stir together the yogurt, cucumber, dill, lemon juice, and garlic until well mixed and season with salt and pepper. Store in a sealed container in the refrigerator for up to 4 days.

COOKING TIP: *The best method to squeeze the juice out of grated cucumber is to pile the grated vegetable in the middle of a clean kitchen cloth, gather up the edges, and twist just above the cucumber to form a pouch. Squeeze the cucumber until the juice comes out, and keep squeezing until the cucumber is basically dry.*

PER SERVING (¼ CUP): *Calories: 28; Total fat: 0g; Saturated fat: 0g; Carbohydrates: 4g; Sugar: 2g; Fiber: 0g; Protein: 4g*

Authentic Baba Ghanoush

SERVES 5 • DAIRY-FREE • GLUTEN-FREE • VEGAN

PREP TIME:
5 MINUTES, PLUS
COOLING TIME

COOK TIME:
40 MINUTES

This is a simple, flavorful, authentic baba ghanoush recipe made with smoky grilled eggplants, tahini, garlic, lemon juice, and olive oil. Baba ghanoush is a Middle Eastern eggplant dip that is full of rich flavor and depth. Eggplant is composed mostly of water and is low in calories, but not only does it have a unique flavor, it boasts significant potassium as well. Serve it with pita bread or fresh vegetables for an easy, healthy snack.

2 extra-large eggplants

3 tablespoons tahini

4 garlic cloves, finely minced

⅓ cup freshly squeezed lemon juice

1 teaspoon sea salt

1 teaspoon olive oil

Dash za'atar spice

Dash sumac spice

1. Preheat the broiler to high. Adjust the oven rack to the middle position and line a baking sheet with aluminum foil.

2. Place the eggplants on the baking sheet and pierce several times with a fork. Broil the eggplants for about 2 minutes on each side, flipping several times to brown the skin on all sides, about 10 minutes.

3. Adjust the oven to 375°F and continue to roast the eggplants for 25 to 30 minutes, until very soft. Remove from the oven and set aside until cool enough to handle, 10 to 15 minutes.

4. While the eggplants are roasting, in a medium bowl, combine the tahini, garlic, lemon juice, and salt.

Continued >

5. Working over a colander, cut the eggplants open and let the liquid drain. Remove and discard the skin.

6. Transfer the drained eggplants to the bowl with the tahini mixture and, using a fork, mash together until a smooth texture is formed. Let cool to room temperature and serve garnished with olive oil, za'atar, and sumac. Store in an airtight container in the refrigerator for up to 5 days.

INGREDIENT TIP: *Za'atar is one of my favorite go-to spice mixes. You can sprinkle it on vegetables, chicken, and beef for an earthy, citrusy flavor. Look for it at specialty markets and online.*

PER SERVING (½ CUP): *Calories: 103; Total fat: 5g; Saturated fat: 1g; Carbohydrates: 13g; Sugar: 6g; Fiber: 7g; Protein: 3g*

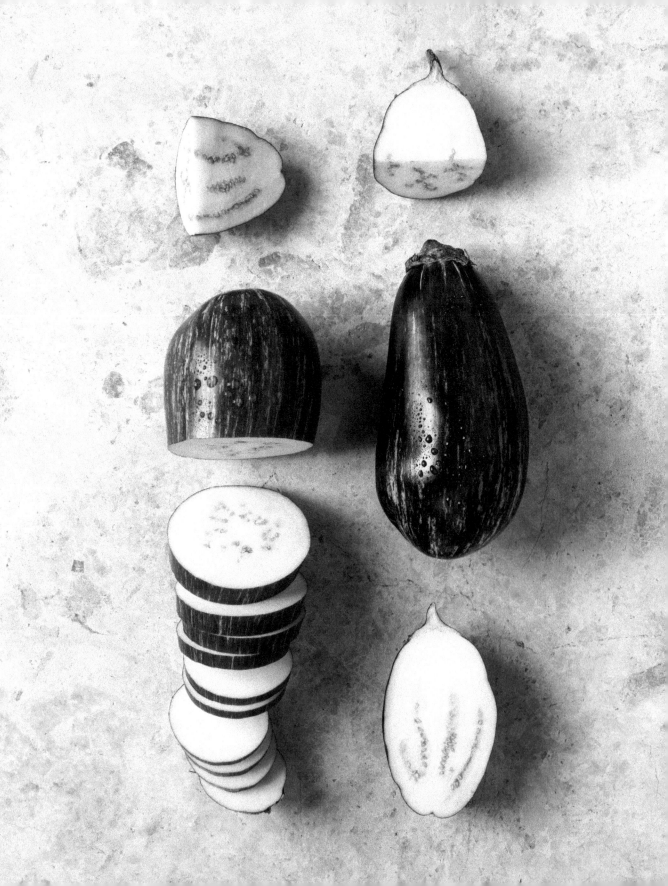

BLANK MEAL PLAN

Make copies of this blank meal plan and use them to plan your meals.

	BREAKFAST	LUNCH	DINNER
MON			
TUE			
WED			
THU			
FRI			
SAT			
SUN			

MEASUREMENT CONVERSIONS

VOLUME EQUIVALENTS (LIQUID)

US Standard	US Standard (ounces)	Metric (approximate)
2 tablespoons	1 fl. oz.	30 mL
¼ cup	2 fl. oz.	60 mL
½ cup	4 fl. oz.	120 mL
1 cup	8 fl. oz.	240 mL
1½ cups	12 fl. oz.	355 mL
2 cups or 1 pint	16 fl. oz.	475 mL
4 cups or 1 quart	32 fl. oz.	1 L
1 gallon	128 fl. oz.	4 L

OVEN TEMPERATURES

Fahrenheit (F)	Celsius (C) (approximate)
250°F	120°C
300°F	150°C
325°F	165°C
350°F	180°C
375°F	190°C
400°F	200°C
425°F	220°C
450°F	230°C

VOLUME EQUIVALENTS (DRY)

US Standard	Metric (approximate)
⅛ teaspoon	0.5 mL
¼ teaspoon	1 mL
½ teaspoon	2 mL
¾ teaspoon	4 mL
1 teaspoon	5 mL
1 tablespoon	15 mL
¼ cup	59 mL
⅓ cup	79 mL
½ cup	118 mL
⅔ cup	156 mL
¾ cup	177 mL
1 cup	235 mL
2 cups or 1 pint	475 mL
3 cups	700 mL
4 cups or 1 quart	1 L

WEIGHT EQUIVALENTS

US Standard	Metric (approximate)
½ ounce	15 g
1 ounce	30 g
2 ounces	60 g
4 ounces	115 g
8 ounces	225 g
12 ounces	340 g
16 ounces or 1 pound	455 g

THE DIRTY DOZEN
AND THE CLEAN FIFTEEN™

A nonprofit environmental watchdog organization called Environmental Working Group (EWG) looks at data supplied by the US Department of Agriculture (USDA) and the Food and Drug Administration (FDA) about pesticide residues. Each year it compiles a list of the best and worst pesticide loads found in commercial crops. You can use these lists to decide which fruits and vegetables to buy organic to minimize your exposure to pesticides and which produce is considered safe enough to buy conventionally. This does not mean they are pesticide-free, though, so wash these fruits and vegetables thoroughly. The list is updated annually, and you can find it online at EWG.org/FoodNews.

DIRTY DOZEN™

1. strawberries
2. spinach
3. kale
4. nectarines
5. apples
6. grapes
7. peaches
8. cherries
9. pears
10. tomatoes
11. celery
12. potatoes

†Additionally, nearly three-quarters of hot pepper samples contained pesticide residues.

CLEAN FIFTEEN™

1. avocados
2. sweet corn
3. pineapples
4. sweet peas (frozen)
5. onions
6. papayas
7. eggplants
8. asparagus
9. kiwis
10. cabbages
11. cauliflower
12. cantaloupes
13. broccoli
14. mushrooms
15. honeydew melons

REFERENCES

American College of Cardiology. "AHA 2019 Heart Disease and Stroke Statistics." February 19, 2019. Accessed May 14, 2019. https://www.acc.org/latest-in-cardiology/ten-points-to-remember /2019/02/15/14/39/aha-2019-heart-disease-and-stroke-statistics.

American Heart Association. "Mediterranean Diet." Accessed May 14, 2019. https://www.heart.org /en/healthy-living/healthy-eating/eat-smart/nutrition-basics/mediterranean-diet.

Global Healthy Living Foundation. "Anti-Inflammatory Diet." Accessed May 1, 2019. https://creakyjoints .org/education/arthritis-diet/anti-inflammatory/?gclid=CjwKCAjw5dnmBRACEiwAmMYGOY 63d2EtCa9ig7fDNuNgkzek89HyifssCE2kvxK2N_qUzR–0TSjrxoCObEQAvD_BwE.

Gonzalez, M.A., and N. Martin-Calvo. "Mediterranean Diet and Life Expectancy; Beyond Olive Oil, Fruits and Vegetables." *Current Opinion in Clinical Nutrition and Metabolic Care* 19, no. 6 (November 2016): 401–407. doi:10.1097/MCO.0000000000000316.

Gunnars, Kris. "Mediterranean Diet 101: A Meal Plan and Beginner's Guide." *Healthline.* July 24, 2018. Accessed May 3, 2019. https://www.healthline.com/nutrition/mediterranean-diet-meal-plan #foods-to-eat.

Harvard T.H. Chan School of Public Health. "Diet Review: Mediterranean Diet." Accessed June 2, 2019. https://www.hsph.harvard.edu/nutritionsource/healthy-weight/diet-reviews/mediterranean-diet/.

Hippocrates Health Institute. "The Benefits of Brocolli Sprouts." Accessed May 14, 2019. https:// hippocratesinst.org/science/brocolli-sprouts.

Keys, Ancel. *Seven Countries: A Multivariate Analysis of Death and Coronary Heart Disease.* Cambridge, MA: Harvard University Press, 2013.

Keys, Ancel, ed. "Coronary Heart Disease in Seven Countries." *Circulation* 41, Suppl. 1 (1970): 1–211.

University Health News. "6 Major Benefits of the Mediterranean Diet." November 2, 2018. Accessed May 1, 2019. https://universityhealthnews.com/daily/nutrition/6-major-benefits-of-the -mediterranean-diet/.

U.S. News and World Report. "Mediterranean Diet: #1 in Best Diets Overall." https://health.usnews .com/best-diet/mediterranean-diet.

Zogheib, Susan. *The Mediterranean Diet Plan: Heart-Healthy Recipes & Meal Plans for Every Type of Eater.* Berkeley, CA: Rockridge Press, 2016.

RECIPE INDEX

A

Asparagus, Apple, and Feta Cheese Omelet, 51–52
Authentic Baba Ghanoush, 193–194
Avocado-Blueberry Smoothie, 96

B

Baked Sardine Patties, 143
Baking Sheet Spicy Shrimp with Vegetables, 108
Balsamic-Basted Beef Kebabs with Barley and
      Spinach Risotto, 33–34
Balsamic Vinegar-Marinated Strawberries, 180
Barley Risotto with Sweet Potato and Spinach, 110
Beet-Fennel Soup with Goat Cheese, 82
Beet-Grapefruit Salad with Citrus-Basil
      Dressing, 78–79
Broiled Flounder with Nectarine and White Bean
      Salsa, 142
Broiled Tomatoes with Feta, 165

C

California Egg White Scramble, 97
Chia-Pomegranate Smoothie, 26
Chicken-Lentil Bowl with Roasted Red Pepper
      Dressing, 150–151
Chicken Shawarma Bowls, 112–113
Chicken with Yogurt-Mint Sauce, 65
Chickpea-Turkey Stew with Spinach, 155–156
Chickpea Veggie Burgers, 109
Chili-Spiced Lamb Chops, 160
Citrus-Artichoke Pesto with Vegetable Noodles, 58
Citrus-Chicken Vegetable "Risotto," 37–38
Citrus-Herb Scallops, 137
Classic Pork Tenderloin Marsala, 157–158
Couscous-Avocado Salad, 176–177
Cranberry-Pumpkin Smoothie, 127
Creamy Panna Cotta, 184

E

Egg-Stuffed Portobello Mushrooms, 129–130
Egg White, Red Pepper, and Chard Scramble,
      73–74

F

Fresh Fruit Crumble Muesli, 71
Fruit-Topped Meringues, 181

G

Goat Cheese, Spinach, and Egg Frittata, 53
Golden Oatmeal Pancakes, 27
Greek Breakfast Tostadas, 131
Greek Herbed Beef Meatballs, 161
Greek Roasted Vegetable Bowl, 64
Greek-Style Tuna Salad in Pita, 100
Greek Vegetable and Herb Pinwheels, 77
Green Vegetable Wrap with Basil Pesto, 31
Grilled Vegetable Open-Faced Sandwich, 32

H

Halibut with Olive-Tomato Sauce, 87
Halibut with Wilted Kale and Cherry Tomatoes, 36
Hummus-Crusted Halibut, 103

K

Kalamata Olive and Sweet Pepper Frittata, 28–29

L

Lemon-Garlic Skillet Chicken, 42–43
Lemon-Spinach Salad with Pears and Blue
      Cheese, 101–102
Light Greek Yogurt Chocolate Pudding, 182
Loaded Smoked Salmon Breakfast Casserole, 75–76

M

Mashed Avocado Egg Salad with Crisps, 171
Mediterranean Romaine Wedge Salad, 172
Moroccan Couscous Salad, 104–105
Moroccan Spiced Chicken with Sweet Potato
      Hash, 88–89

N

North African Chicken Apricot Tagine, 106–107

O

Oatmeal Bowls with Blackberries, Seeds, and
      Honey, 124–125
Oven-Roasted Puttanesca with Ground Beef, 56–57
Overnight Steel-Cut Oats Porridge with Cherries, 95

P

Pan-Fried Chicken with Roasted Squash
      Salsa, 148–149

Parmesan-Sautéed Zucchini with Spaghetti, 166
Pesto Vinaigrette, 190
Pomegranate Granita, 183

Q

Quinoa and Spinach Salad with Figs and Balsamic
    Dressing, 30
Quinoa Nuts and Seeds Overnight Porridge, 25
Quinoa-Walnut Pancakes, 128

R

Roasted Brussels Sprouts and Halloumi
    Salad, 173–174
Roasted Garlic, 189
Roasted Vegetable Mélange, 175
Rosemary-Citrus Roasted Pork Tenderloin, 159
Skillet Cod with Fresh Tomato Salsa, 141

S

Salmon, Citrus, and Avocado Salad, 54
Salmon Bowl with Bulgur and Tahini Sauce, 85–86
Salmon Provençal, 144
Sautéed Dark Leafy Greens, 164
Savory Hummus Breakfast Toasts, 50
Shaved Cucumber Quinoa Bowl, 41
Simple Bouillabaisse, 39–40
Sirloin with Sweet Bell Peppers, 83
Skillet Chicken Thighs with Bulgur and Feta,
    152–153
Speedy Marinara Sauce, 191

Spiced Oranges with Dates, 185
Spicy Broccoli-Shrimp Farfalle, 138–139
Spicy Split Pea Tabbouleh, 170
Stone Fruit Overnight Bulgur, 72
Strawberry and Brown Rice Sunflower Seed Bowl, 126
Sun-dried Tomato and Olive Tapenade with Goat
    Cheese Toasts, 55
Sun-dried Tomato and Asparagus Frittata, 98–99
Sweet Kale Smoothie, 49

T

Tabbouleh Pita Sandwich, 84
Tomato and Lentil Soup, 35
Tomato and Wine-Steamed Mussels, 136
Tomato-Asparagus Omelets, 132–133
Tomatoes Stuffed with Herbed Bulgur, 59–60
Traditional Falafel, 168–169
Traditional Hummus, 188
Trout with Roasted Red Pepper Sauce, 63
Trout with Ruby Red Grapefruit Relish, 145
Tuna Couscous Bowl with Grilled Vegetables, 61–62
Tunisian Herb Chicken Skewers, 111
Turkey-Tomato Ragù, 154
Tzatziki Sauce, 192

W

Whole Baked Trout with Lemon and Herbs, 140
Whole-Wheat Spaghetti with Shrimp and Mint
    Pesto, 80–81
Wild Rice with Grapes, 167

INDEX

A

Almonds
  Fresh Fruit Crumble Muesli, 71
  Overnight Steel-Cut Oats Porridge with
    Cherries, 95
  Roasted Brussels Sprouts and Halloumi Salad,
    173–174
American Heart Association (AHA), 4
Apples
  Asparagus, Apple, and Feta Cheese Omelet,
    51–52
  Sweet Kale Smoothie, 49
Apricots, dried
  Moroccan Couscous Salad, 104–105
  North African Chicken Apricot Tagine,
    106–107
Artichoke hearts
  Chicken-Lentil Bowl with Roasted Red Pepper
    Dressing, 150–151
  Citrus-Artichoke Pesto with Vegetable
    Noodles, 58
  Couscous-Avocado Salad, 176–177
  Greek Breakfast Tostadas, 131
  Greek Roasted Vegetable Bowl, 64
Arugula
  Roasted Brussels Sprouts and Halloumi Salad,
    173–174
Asiago cheese
  Citrus-Artichoke Pesto with Vegetable
    Noodles, 58
  Mediterranean Romaine Wedge Salad, 172
Asparagus
  Asparagus, Apple, and Feta Cheese Omelet,
    51–52
  Baking Sheet Spicy Shrimp with Vegetables, 108
  Sun-dried Tomato and Asparagus Frittata,
    98–99
  Tomato-Asparagus Omelets, 132–133
Avocados
  Avocado-Blueberry Smoothie, 96
  California Egg White Scramble, 97
  Couscous-Avocado Salad, 176–177
  Mashed Avocado Egg Salad with Crisps, 171
  Salmon, Citrus, and Avocado Salad, 54

B

Barley, pearled
  Balsamic-Basted Beef Kebabs with Barley and
    Spinach Risotto, 33–34
  Barley Risotto with Sweet Potato and
    Spinach, 110
Basil
  Asparagus, Apple, and Feta Cheese Omelet, 51–52
  Beet-Grapefruit Salad with Citrus-Basil Dressing,
    78–79
  Broiled Tomatoes with Feta, 165
  California Egg White Scramble, 97
  Chicken-Lentil Bowl with Roasted Red Pepper
    Dressing, 150–151
  Citrus-Artichoke Pesto with Vegetable
    Noodles, 58
  Greek Breakfast Tostadas, 131
  Greek Roasted Vegetable Bowl, 64
  Greek Vegetable and Herb Pinwheels, 77
  Green Vegetable Wrap with Basil Pesto, 31
  Halibut with Wilted Kale and Cherry Tomatoes, 36
  Mediterranean Romaine Wedge Salad, 172
  Oven-Roasted Puttanesca with Ground Beef, 56–57
  Skillet Cod with Fresh Tomato Salsa, 141
  Speedy Marinara Sauce, 191
  Sun-dried Tomato and Asparagus Frittata, 98–99
  Tomato and Lentil Soup, 35
  Tomato-Asparagus Omelets, 132–133
  Tomatoes Stuffed with Herbed Bulgur, 59–60
  Turkey-Tomato Ragù, 154
  Whole-Wheat Spaghetti with Shrimp and Mint
    Pesto, 80–81
Beans and legumes, 7, 9, 16. See also specific
Beef
  Balsamic-Basted Beef Kebabs with Barley and
    Spinach Risotto, 33–34
  Greek Herbed Beef Meatballs, 161
  Oven-Roasted Puttanesca with Ground Beef,
    56–57
  Sirloin with Sweet Bell Peppers, 83
Beets
  Beet-Fennel Soup with Goat Cheese, 82
  Beet-Grapefruit Salad with Citrus-Basil Dressing,
    78–79

Berries
    Avocado-Blueberry Smoothie, 96
    Balsamic Vinegar-Marinated Strawberries, 180
    Chia-Pomegranate Smoothie, 26
    Creamy Panna Cotta, 184
    Fresh Fruit Crumble Muesli, 71
    Fruit-Topped Meringues, 181
    Lemon-Spinach Salad with Pears and Blue Cheese, 101–102
    Oatmeal Bowls with Blackberries, Seeds, and Honey, 124–125
    Roasted Brussels Sprouts and Halloumi Salad, 173–174
    Strawberry and Brown Rice Sunflower Seed Bowl, 126
Blood glucose, 4, 6
Blue cheese
    Lemon-Spinach Salad with Pears and Blue Cheese, 101–102
Bok choy
    Baking Sheet Spicy Shrimp with Vegetables, 108
Bowls
    building, 118
    Chicken-Lentil Bowl with Roasted Red Pepper Dressing, 150–151
    Greek Roasted Vegetable Bowl, 64
    Oatmeal Bowls with Blackberries, Seeds, and Honey, 124–125
    Salmon Bowl with Bulgur and Tahini Sauce, 85–86
    Shaved Cucumber Quinoa Bowl, 41
    Strawberry and Brown Rice Sunflower Seed Bowl, 126
    Tuna Couscous Bowl with Grilled Vegetables, 61–62
Brain function, 6
Breakfast builder, 117
Broccoli
    Loaded Smoked Salmon Breakfast Casserole, 75–76
    Moroccan Couscous Salad, 104–105
    Roasted Vegetable Mélange, 175
    Shaved Cucumber Quinoa Bowl, 41
    Spicy Broccoli-Shrimp Farfalle, 138–139
Brussels sprouts
    Roasted Brussels Sprouts and Halloumi Salad, 173–174
Bulgur
    Salmon Bowl with Bulgur and Tahini Sauce, 85–86
    Skillet Chicken Thighs with Bulgur and Feta, 152–153
    Stone Fruit Overnight Bulgur, 72
    Tomatoes Stuffed with Herbed Bulgur, 59–60

C
Cannellini beans
    Broiled Flounder with Nectarine and White Bean Salsa, 142
Carrots
    Chickpea-Turkey Stew with Spinach, 155–156
    Chickpea Veggie Burgers, 109
    Citrus-Chicken Vegetable "Risotto," 37–38
    Greek Roasted Vegetable Bowl, 64
    Greek Vegetable and Herb Pinwheels, 77
    Moroccan Couscous Salad, 104–105
    North African Chicken Apricot Tagine, 106–107
    Savory Hummus Breakfast Toasts, 50
Cauliflower
    Citrus-Chicken Vegetable "Risotto," 37–38
    North African Chicken Apricot Tagine, 106–107
    Roasted Vegetable Mélange, 175
Celery root
    Greek Roasted Vegetable Bowl, 64
Cheese. *See specific*
Cherries
    Overnight Steel-Cut Oats Porridge with Cherries, 95
    Stone Fruit Overnight Bulgur, 72
Chia seeds
    Chia-Pomegranate Smoothie, 26
    Overnight Steel-Cut Oats Porridge with Cherries, 95
Chicken, 7, 9
    Chicken-Lentil Bowl with Roasted Red Pepper Dressing, 150–151
    Chicken Shawarma Bowls, 112–113
    Chicken with Yogurt-Mint Sauce, 65
    Citrus-Chicken Vegetable "Risotto," 37–38
    Lemon-Garlic Skillet Chicken, 42–43
    Moroccan Spiced Chicken with Sweet Potato Hash, 88–89
    North African Chicken Apricot Tagine, 106–107
    Pan-Fried Chicken with Roasted Squash Salsa, 148–149
    Skillet Chicken Thighs with Bulgur and Feta, 152–153
    Tunisian Herb Chicken Skewers, 111
Chickpeas
    Chicken Shawarma Bowls, 112–113
    Chickpea-Turkey Stew with Spinach, 155–156
    Chickpea Veggie Burgers, 109
    Traditional Falafel, 168–169
    Traditional Hummus, 188
Chocolate
    Light Greek Yogurt Chocolate Pudding, 182

Cilantro
> Broiled Flounder with Nectarine and White Bean Salsa, 142
> California Egg White Scramble, 97
> Chickpea-Turkey Stew with Spinach, 155–156
> Chili-Spiced Lamb Chops, 160
> Citrus-Herb Scallops, 137
> Spicy Split Pea Tabbouleh, 170
> Traditional Falafel, 168–169

Coconut
> Strawberry and Brown Rice Sunflower Seed Bowl, 126

Cod
> Skillet Cod with Fresh Tomato Salsa, 141

Cottage cheese
> Golden Oatmeal Pancakes, 27

Couscous
> Couscous-Avocado Salad, 176–177
> Moroccan Couscous Salad, 104–105
> Tuna Couscous Bowl with Grilled Vegetables, 61–62

Cranberry juice
> Cranberry-Pumpkin Smoothie, 127

Cucumbers
> Chicken-Lentil Bowl with Roasted Red Pepper Dressing, 150–151
> Chicken Shawarma Bowls, 112–113
> Couscous-Avocado Salad, 176–177
> Greek-Style Tuna Salad in Pita, 100
> Green Vegetable Wrap with Basil Pesto, 31
> Mediterranean Romaine Wedge Salad, 172
> Savory Hummus Breakfast Toasts, 50
> Shaved Cucumber Quinoa Bowl, 41
> Spicy Split Pea Tabbouleh, 170
> Tabbouleh Pita Sandwich, 84
> Trout with Ruby Red Grapefruit Relish, 145
> Tzatziki Sauce, 192

D

Dairy-free
> Authentic Baba Ghanoush, 193–194
> Baked Sardine Patties, 143
> Baking Sheet Spicy Shrimp with Vegetables, 108
> Balsamic-Basted Beef Kebabs with Barley and Spinach Risotto, 33–34
> Balsamic Vinegar-Marinated Strawberries, 180
> Broiled Flounder with Nectarine and White Bean Salsa, 142
> California Egg White Scramble, 97
> Chia-Pomegranate Smoothie, 26
> Chicken-Lentil Bowl with Roasted Red Pepper Dressing, 150–151

Chickpea-Turkey Stew with Spinach, 155–156
Chickpea Veggie Burgers, 109
Chili-Spiced Lamb Chops, 160
Citrus-Herb Scallops, 137
Classic Pork Tenderloin Marsala, 157–158
Cranberry-Pumpkin Smoothie, 127
Egg-Stuffed Portobello Mushrooms, 129–130
Egg White, Red Pepper, and Chard Scramble, 73–74
Fruit-Topped Meringues, 181
Greek Roasted Vegetable Bowl, 64
Halibut with Olive-Tomato Sauce, 87
Halibut with Wilted Kale and Cherry Tomatoes, 36
Hummus-Crusted Halibut, 103
Lemon-Garlic Skillet Chicken, 42–43
Loaded Smoked Salmon Breakfast Casserole, 75–76
Mashed Avocado Egg Salad with Crisps, 171
Moroccan Couscous Salad, 104–105
Moroccan Spiced Chicken with Sweet Potato Hash, 88–89
North African Chicken Apricot Tagine, 106–107
Oatmeal Bowls with Blackberries, Seeds, and Honey, 124–125
Overnight Steel-Cut Oats Porridge with Cherries, 95
Pan-Fried Chicken with Roasted Squash Salsa, 148–149
Pesto Vinaigrette, 190
Pomegranate Granita, 183
Quinoa Nuts and Seeds Overnight Porridge, 25
Quinoa-Walnut Pancakes, 128
Roasted Vegetable Mélange, 175
Rosemary-Citrus Roasted Pork Tenderloin, 159
Salmon, Citrus, and Avocado Salad, 54
Salmon Bowl with Bulgur and Tahini Sauce, 85–86
Salmon Provençal, 144
Sautéed Dark Leafy Greens, 164
Shaved Cucumber Quinoa Bowl, 41
Simple Bouillabaisse, 39–40
Sirloin with Sweet Bell Peppers, 83
Skillet Cod with Fresh Tomato Salsa, 141
Speedy Marinara Sauce, 191
Spiced Oranges with Dates, 185
Spicy Broccoli-Shrimp Farfalle, 138–139
Spicy Split Pea Tabbouleh, 170
Strawberry and Brown Rice Sunflower Seed Bowl, 126
Tomato and Lentil Soup, 35
Tomato and Wine-Steamed Mussels, 136
Tomato-Asparagus Omelets, 132–133

Dairy-free *(continued)*
  Tomatoes Stuffed with Herbed Bulgur, 59–60
  Traditional Falafel, 168–169
  Traditional Hummus, 188
  Trout with Roasted Red Pepper Sauce, 63
  Trout with Ruby Red Grapefruit Relish, 145
  Tuna Couscous Bowl with Grilled Vegetables,
    61–62
  Tunisian Herb Chicken Skewers, 111
  Turkey-Tomato Ragù, 154
  Whole Baked Trout with Lemon and Herbs, 140
  Wild Rice with Grapes, 167
Dairy products, 7, 9
Dates, 16
  Chia-Pomegranate Smoothie, 26
  Fresh Fruit Crumble Muesli, 71
  Spiced Oranges with Dates, 185
  Sweet Kale Smoothie, 49
Desserts. *See* Sweets
Diabetes, 4, 6
Digestion, 6
Dill
  Baked Sardine Patties, 143
  Chicken with Yogurt-Mint Sauce, 65
  Loaded Smoked Salmon Breakfast Casserole,
    75–76
  Tzatziki Sauce, 192
  Whole Baked Trout with Lemon and Herbs, 140
Dips and Spreads. *See also* Salsas
  Authentic Baba Ghanoush, 193–194
  Roasted Garlic, 189
  Traditional Hummus, 188
Dressings
  Citrus-Basil Dressing, 78–79
  Pesto Vinaigrette, 190
  Roasted Red Pepper Dressing, 150–151

E

Eating out, 119
Edamame
  Salmon Bowl with Bulgur and Tahini Sauce, 85–86
Eggplants
  Authentic Baba Ghanoush, 193–194
  Tuna Couscous Bowl with Grilled Vegetables,
    61–62
Eggs, 7, 16
  Asparagus, Apple, and Feta Cheese Omelet,
    51–52
  Baked Sardine Patties, 143
  California Egg White Scramble, 97
  Egg-Stuffed Portobello Mushrooms, 129–130
  Egg White, Red Pepper, and Chard Scramble, 73–74
  Fruit-Topped Meringues, 181
  Goat Cheese, Spinach, and Egg Frittata, 53
  Greek Breakfast Tostadas, 131
  Greek Herbed Beef Meatballs, 161
  Kalamata Olive and Sweet Pepper Frittata, 28–29
  Loaded Smoked Salmon Breakfast Casserole,
    75–76
  Mashed Avocado Egg Salad with Crisps, 171
  Quinoa-Walnut Pancakes, 128
  Sun-dried Tomato and Asparagus Frittata, 98–99
  Tomato-Asparagus Omelets, 132–133
Equipment, 14–15
Exercise, 10–11

F

Fats, healthy, 7, 9
Fennel
  Beet-Fennel Soup with Goat Cheese, 82
  Mediterranean Romaine Wedge Salad, 172
  Simple Bouillabaisse, 39–40
Feta cheese
  Asparagus, Apple, and Feta Cheese Omelet,
    51–52
  Broiled Tomatoes with Feta, 165
  Couscous-Avocado Salad, 176–177
  Greek-Style Tuna Salad in Pita, 100
  Green Vegetable Wrap with Basil Pesto, 31
  Grilled Vegetable Open-Faced Sandwich, 32
  Savory Hummus Breakfast Toasts, 50
  Skillet Chicken Thighs with Bulgur and Feta,
    152–153
Figs
  Quinoa and Spinach Salad with Figs and Balsamic
    Dressing, 30
Fish, 7, 9, 16
  Baked Sardine Patties, 143
  Broiled Flounder with Nectarine and White Bean
    Salsa, 142
  Greek-Style Tuna Salad in Pita, 100
  Halibut with Olive-Tomato Sauce, 87
  Halibut with Wilted Kale and Cherry Tomatoes, 36
  Hummus-Crusted Halibut, 103
  Loaded Smoked Salmon Breakfast Casserole,
    75–76
  Skillet Cod with Fresh Tomato Salsa, 141
  Salmon, Citrus, and Avocado Salad, 54
  Salmon Bowl with Bulgur and Tahini Sauce, 85–86
  Salmon Provençal, 144
  Simple Bouillabaisse, 39–40
  Trout with Roasted Red Pepper Sauce, 63

Trout with Ruby Red Grapefruit Relish, 145

Tuna Couscous Bowl with Grilled Vegetables, 61–62

Whole Baked Trout with Lemon and Herbs, 140

Flaxseed

Oatmeal Bowls with Blackberries, Seeds, and Honey, 124–125

Flounder

Broiled Flounder with Nectarine and White Bean Salsa, 142

Food swaps, 8

Freezer staples, 17

Fruits, 6, 9, 17. *See also specific*

G

Garlic, 16

Lemon-Garlic Skillet Chicken, 42–43

Roasted Garlic, 189

Gluten-free

Authentic Baba Ghanoush, 193–194

Avocado-Blueberry Smoothie, 96

Baking Sheet Spicy Shrimp with Vegetables, 108

Balsamic Vinegar-Marinated Strawberries, 180

Beet-Fennel Soup with Goat Cheese, 82

Beet-Grapefruit Salad with Citrus-Basil Dressing, 78–79

Broiled Flounder with Nectarine and White Bean Salsa, 142

Broiled Tomatoes with Feta, 165

California Egg White Scramble, 97

Chia-Pomegranate Smoothie, 26

Chicken-Lentil Bowl with Roasted Red Pepper Dressing, 150–151

Chicken Shawarma Bowls, 112–113

Chicken with Yogurt-Mint Sauce, 65

Chickpea-Turkey Stew with Spinach, 155–156

Chili-Spiced Lamb Chops, 160

Citrus-Chicken Vegetable "Risotto," 37–38

Citrus-Herb Scallops, 137

Cranberry-Pumpkin Smoothie, 127

Creamy Panna Cotta, 184

Egg-Stuffed Portobello Mushrooms, 129–130

Egg White, Red Pepper, and Chard Scramble, 73–74

Fresh Fruit Crumble Muesli, 71

Fruit-Topped Meringues, 181

Goat Cheese, Spinach, and Egg Frittata, 53

Golden Oatmeal Pancakes, 27

Greek Breakfast Tostadas, 131

Greek Roasted Vegetable Bowl, 64

Halibut with Olive-Tomato Sauce, 87

Halibut with Wilted Kale and Cherry Tomatoes, 36

Kalamata Olive and Sweet Pepper Frittata, 28–29

Lemon-Garlic Skillet Chicken, 42–43

Lemon-Spinach Salad with Pears and Blue Cheese, 101–102

Light Greek Yogurt Chocolate Pudding, 182

Loaded Smoked Salmon Breakfast Casserole, 75–76

Mediterranean Romaine Wedge Salad, 172

Moroccan Spiced Chicken with Sweet Potato Hash, 88–89

North African Chicken Apricot Tagine, 106–107

Oatmeal Bowls with Blackberries, Seeds, and Honey, 124–125

Overnight Steel-Cut Oats Porridge with Cherries, 95

Pan-Fried Chicken with Roasted Squash Salsa, 148–149

Pesto Vinaigrette, 190

Pomegranate Granita, 183

Quinoa and Spinach Salad with Figs and Balsamic Dressing, 30

Quinoa Nuts and Seeds Overnight Porridge, 25

Roasted Brussels Sprouts and Halloumi Salad, 173–174

Skillet Cod with Fresh Tomato Salsa, 141

Roasted Garlic, 189

Roasted Vegetable Mélange, 175

Rosemary-Citrus Roasted Pork Tenderloin, 159

Salmon, Citrus, and Avocado Salad, 54

Salmon Provençal, 144

Sautéed Dark Leafy Greens, 164

Shaved Cucumber Quinoa Bowl, 41

Simple Bouillabaisse, 39–40

Sirloin with Sweet Bell Peppers, 83

Speedy Marinara Sauce, 191

Spiced Oranges with Dates, 185

Spicy Split Pea Tabbouleh, 170

Strawberry and Brown Rice Sunflower Seed Bowl, 126

Sun-dried Tomato and Asparagus Frittata, 98–99

Sweet Kale Smoothie, 49

Tomato and Lentil Soup, 35

Tomato and Wine-Steamed Mussels, 136

Tomato-Asparagus Omelets, 132–133

Traditional Hummus, 188

Trout with Roasted Red Pepper Sauce, 63

Trout with Ruby Red Grapefruit Relish, 145

Tunisian Herb Chicken Skewers, 111

Tzatziki Sauce, 192

Whole Baked Trout with Lemon and Herbs, 140

Wild Rice with Grapes, 167

Goat cheese
  Beet-Fennel Soup with Goat Cheese, 82
  Beet-Grapefruit Salad with Citrus-Basil Dressing,
    78–79
  Goat Cheese, Spinach, and Egg Frittata, 53
  Kalamata Olive and Sweet Pepper Frittata, 28–29
  Quinoa and Spinach Salad with Figs and Balsamic
    Dressing, 30
  Sun-dried Tomato and Olive Tapenade with Goat
    Cheese Toasts, 55
Grapefruits
  Beet-Grapefruit Salad with Citrus-Basil Dressing,
    78–79
  Salmon, Citrus, and Avocado Salad, 54
  Trout with Ruby Red Grapefruit Relish, 145
Grapes
  Wild Rice with Grapes, 167
Green beans
  Green Vegetable Wrap with Basil Pesto, 31
  Tomatoes Stuffed with Herbed Bulgur, 59–60
  Whole-Wheat Spaghetti with Shrimp and Mint
    Pesto, 80–81
Greens, leafy, 15. See also specific
  Beet-Grapefruit Salad with Citrus-Basil Dressing,
    78–79
  Salmon, Citrus, and Avocado Salad, 54
  Sautéed Dark Leafy Greens, 164

H
Halibut
  Halibut with Olive-Tomato Sauce, 87
  Halibut with Wilted Kale and Cherry
    Tomatoes, 36
  Hummus-Crusted Halibut, 103
Halloumi cheese
  Roasted Brussels Sprouts and Halloumi Salad,
    173–174
Hazelnuts
  Spiced Oranges with Dates, 185
Heart disease, 4
Herbs, 7, 16–17
Honey, 16
Hummus
  Greek Breakfast Tostadas, 131
  Hummus-Crusted Halibut, 103
  Savory Hummus Breakfast Toasts, 50
  Traditional Hummus, 188

I
Inflammation, 6

K
Kale
  Chia-Pomegranate Smoothie, 26
  Chicken-Lentil Bowl with Roasted Red Pepper
    Dressing, 150–151
  Halibut with Wilted Kale and Cherry Tomatoes, 36
  Moroccan Spiced Chicken with Sweet Potato
    Hash, 88–89
  Salmon Provençal, 144
  Simple Bouillabaisse, 39–40
  Sweet Kale Smoothie, 49
Keys, Ancel, 4
Kiwis
  Fresh Fruit Crumble Muesli, 71

L
Lamb
  Chili-Spiced Lamb Chops, 160
Leftovers, 117
Lemons
  Authentic Baba Ghanoush, 193–194
  Baked Sardine Patties, 143
  Chicken Shawarma Bowls, 112–113
  Chickpea-Turkey Stew with Spinach, 155–156
  Citrus-Artichoke Pesto with Vegetable
    Noodles, 58
  Citrus-Chicken Vegetable "Risotto," 37–38
  Greek Roasted Vegetable Bowl, 64
  Greek-Style Tuna Salad in Pita, 100
  Halibut with Wilted Kale and Cherry Tomatoes, 36
  Lemon-Garlic Skillet Chicken, 42–43
  Lemon-Spinach Salad with Pears and Blue Cheese,
    101–102
  Mashed Avocado Egg Salad with Crisps, 171
  Pan-Fried Chicken with Roasted Squash Salsa,
    148–149
  Roasted Brussels Sprouts and Halloumi Salad,
    173–174
  Rosemary-Citrus Roasted Pork Tenderloin, 159
  Salmon Bowl with Bulgur and Tahini Sauce, 85–86
  Sautéed Dark Leafy Greens, 164
  Sirloin with Sweet Bell Peppers, 83
  Skillet Chicken Thighs with Bulgur and Feta,
    152–153
  Spicy Broccoli-Shrimp Farfalle, 138–139
  Sun-dried Tomato and Olive Tapenade with Goat
    Cheese Toasts, 55
  Sweet Kale Smoothie, 49
  Tabbouleh Pita Sandwich, 84
  Tomato and Wine-Steamed Mussels, 136

Tomatoes Stuffed with Herbed Bulgur, 59–60
Traditional Falafel, 168–169
Traditional Hummus, 188
Trout with Roasted Red Pepper Sauce, 63
Tuna Couscous Bowl with Grilled Vegetables,
    61–62
Tunisian Herb Chicken Skewers, 111
Tzatziki Sauce, 192
Whole Baked Trout with Lemon and Herbs, 140
Lentils
    Chicken-Lentil Bowl with Roasted Red Pepper
        Dressing, 150–151
    Moroccan Couscous Salad, 104–105
    Tomato and Lentil Soup, 35
Lettuce
    Greek-Style Tuna Salad in Pita, 100
    Mediterranean Romaine Wedge Salad, 172
    Salmon Bowl with Bulgur and Tahini Sauce, 85–86
Limes
    Baking Sheet Spicy Shrimp with Vegetables, 108
    Beet-Grapefruit Salad with Citrus-Basil Dressing,
        78–79
    Broiled Flounder with Nectarine and White Bean
        Salsa, 142
    Citrus-Herb Scallops, 137
    Moroccan Couscous Salad, 104–105
    Rosemary-Citrus Roasted Pork Tenderloin, 159
    Spicy Split Pea Tabbouleh, 170
    Trout with Ruby Red Grapefruit Relish, 145
    Whole-Wheat Spaghetti with Shrimp and Mint
        Pesto, 80–81

M
Meal in one
    Avocado-Blueberry Smoothie, 96
    Baking Sheet Spicy Shrimp with Vegetables, 108
    Balsamic-Basted Beef Kebabs with Barley and
        Spinach Risotto, 33–34
    Barley Risotto with Sweet Potato and
        Spinach, 110
    Beet-Fennel Soup with Goat Cheese, 82
    Beet-Grapefruit Salad with Citrus-Basil Dressing,
        78–79
    California Egg White Scramble, 97
    Chia-Pomegranate Smoothie, 26
    Chicken-Lentil Bowl with Roasted Red Pepper
        Dressing, 150–151
    Chicken Shawarma Bowls, 112–113
    Chicken with Yogurt-Mint Sauce, 65
    Chickpea-Turkey Stew with Spinach, 155–156

Citrus-Chicken Vegetable "Risotto," 37–38
Couscous-Avocado Salad, 176–177
Cranberry-Pumpkin Smoothie, 127
Egg-Stuffed Portobello Mushrooms, 129–130
Egg White, Red Pepper, and Chard Scramble,
    73–74
Fresh Fruit Crumble Muesli, 71
Goat Cheese, Spinach, and Egg Frittata, 53
Golden Oatmeal Pancakes, 27
Greek Breakfast Tostadas, 131
Greek Roasted Vegetable Bowl, 64
Greek-Style Tuna Salad in Pita, 100
Greek Vegetable and Herb Pinwheels, 77
Green Vegetable Wrap with Basil Pesto, 31
Grilled Vegetable Open-Faced Sandwich, 32
Halibut with Wilted Kale and Cherry Tomatoes, 36
Kalamata Olive and Sweet Pepper Frittata, 28–29
Lemon-Spinach Salad with Pears and Blue Cheese,
    101–102
Loaded Smoked Salmon Breakfast Casserole,
    75–76
Mashed Avocado Egg Salad with Crisps, 171
Mediterranean Romaine Wedge Salad, 172
Moroccan Couscous Salad, 104–105
Moroccan Spiced Chicken with Sweet Potato
    Hash, 88–89
North African Chicken Apricot Tagine, 106–107
Oatmeal Bowls with Blackberries, Seeds, and
    Honey, 124–125
Oven-Roasted Puttanesca with Ground Beef,
    56–57
Overnight Steel-Cut Oats Porridge with
    Cherries, 95
Quinoa and Spinach Salad with Figs and Balsamic
    Dressing, 30
Quinoa Nuts and Seeds Overnight Porridge, 25
Quinoa-Walnut Pancakes, 128
Roasted Brussels Sprouts and Halloumi Salad,
    173–174
Roasted Vegetable Mélange, 175
Salmon, Citrus, and Avocado Salad, 54
Salmon Bowl with Bulgur and Tahini Sauce,
    85–86
Savory Hummus Breakfast Toasts, 50
Shaved Cucumber Quinoa Bowl, 41
Simple Bouillabaisse, 39–40
Skillet Chicken Thighs with Bulgur and Feta,
    152–153
Spicy Broccoli-Shrimp Farfalle, 138–139
Spicy Split Pea Tabbouleh, 170

Meal in one *(continued)*
    Stone Fruit Overnight Bulgur, 72
    Strawberry and Brown Rice Sunflower Seed
        Bowl, 126
    Sun-dried Tomato and Asparagus Frittata, 98–99
    Sun-dried Tomato and Olive Tapenade with Goat
        Cheese Toasts, 55
    Sweet Kale Smoothie, 49
    Tabbouleh Pita Sandwich, 84
    Tomato and Lentil Soup, 35
    Tomato and Wine-Steamed Mussels, 136
    Tomato-Asparagus Omelets, 132–133
    Traditional Falafel, 168–169
    Tuna Couscous Bowl with Grilled Vegetables,
        61–62
    Turkey-Tomato Ragù, 154
    Whole Baked Trout with Lemon and Herbs, 140
    Whole-Wheat Spaghetti with Shrimp and Mint
        Pesto, 80–81
Meal planning
    tips, 116
    week one, 21–24
    week two, 45–48
    week three, 67–70
    week four, 91–94
Mealtimes, 10
Meats, 8
Mediterranean diet
    about, 4
    benefits of, 4, 6, 11
    food swaps, 8
    lifestyle changes, 10–11
    plating, 9
    pyramid, 5
Mint
    Chicken with Yogurt-Mint Sauce, 65
    Moroccan Couscous Salad, 104–105
    Whole-Wheat Spaghetti with Shrimp and Mint
        Pesto, 80–81
Mood, 6
Mozzarella cheese
    Greek Breakfast Tostadas, 131
    Sun-dried Tomato and Asparagus Frittata, 98–99
Mushrooms
    Classic Pork Tenderloin Marsala, 157–158
    Egg-Stuffed Portobello Mushrooms, 129–130
    Roasted Vegetable Mélange, 175
Mussels
    Simple Bouillabaisse, 39–40
    Tomato and Wine-Steamed Mussels, 136

N
Nectarines
    Broiled Flounder with Nectarine and White Bean
        Salsa, 142
    Fresh Fruit Crumble Muesli, 71
Nuts, 7, 9, 16. *See also specific*

O
Oats
    Avocado-Blueberry Smoothie, 96
    Fresh Fruit Crumble Muesli, 71
    Golden Oatmeal Pancakes, 27
    Oatmeal Bowls with Blackberries, Seeds, and
        Honey, 124–125
    Overnight Steel-Cut Oats Porridge with
        Cherries, 95
    Quinoa Nuts and Seeds Overnight Porridge, 25
Olive oil, 15
Olives, black
    Salmon Provençal, 144
Olives, green
    Shaved Cucumber Quinoa Bowl, 41
    Skillet Cod with Fresh Tomato Salsa, 141
Olives, Kalamata
    Greek Roasted Vegetable Bowl, 64
    Greek-Style Tuna Salad in Pita, 100
    Halibut with Olive-Tomato Sauce, 87
    Kalamata Olive and Sweet Pepper Frittata,
        28–29
    Mediterranean Romaine Wedge Salad, 172
    Oven-Roasted Puttanesca with Ground Beef,
        56–57
    Savory Hummus Breakfast Toasts, 50
    Skillet Chicken Thighs with Bulgur and Feta,
        152–153
    Sun-dried Tomato and Olive Tapenade with Goat
        Cheese Toasts, 55
    Tomato and Wine-Steamed Mussels, 136
Oranges
    Beet-Grapefruit Salad with Citrus-Basil Dressing,
        78–79
    Salmon, Citrus, and Avocado Salad, 54
    Spiced Oranges with Dates, 185
    Trout with Ruby Red Grapefruit Relish, 145

P
Pancakes
    Golden Oatmeal Pancakes, 27
    Quinoa-Walnut Pancakes, 128
Pantry staples, 15–16

Parmesan cheese
    Barley Risotto with Sweet Potato and Spinach, 110
    Citrus-Chicken Vegetable "Risotto," 37–38
    Greek Herbed Beef Meatballs, 161
    Oven-Roasted Puttanesca with Ground Beef, 56–57
    Parmesan-Sautéed Zucchini with Spaghetti, 166
    Whole-Wheat Spaghetti with Shrimp and Mint Pesto, 80–81
Parsnips
    Greek Roasted Vegetable Bowl, 64
Pasta
    Oven-Roasted Puttanesca with Ground Beef, 56–57
    Parmesan-Sautéed Zucchini with Spaghetti, 166
    Spicy Broccoli-Shrimp Farfalle, 138–139
    Turkey-Tomato Ragù, 154
    Whole-Wheat Spaghetti with Shrimp and Mint Pesto, 80–81
Peaches
    Stone Fruit Overnight Bulgur, 72
Pears
    Lemon-Spinach Salad with Pears and Blue Cheese, 101–102
    Pan-Fried Chicken with Roasted Squash Salsa, 148–149
Pecans
    Beet-Grapefruit Salad with Citrus-Basil Dressing, 78–79
    Fresh Fruit Crumble Muesli, 71
    Quinoa Nuts and Seeds Overnight Porridge, 25
    Salmon, Citrus, and Avocado Salad, 54
    Stone Fruit Overnight Bulgur, 72
Peppers, bell
    Baking Sheet Spicy Shrimp with Vegetables, 108
    Balsamic-Basted Beef Kebabs with Barley and Spinach Risotto, 33–34
    Broiled Flounder with Nectarine and White Bean Salsa, 142
    Citrus-Chicken Vegetable "Risotto," 37–38
    Egg-Stuffed Portobello Mushrooms, 129–130
    Egg White, Red Pepper, and Chard Scramble, 73–74
    Greek-Style Tuna Salad in Pita, 100
    Greek Vegetable and Herb Pinwheels, 77
    Green Vegetable Wrap with Basil Pesto, 31
    Kalamata Olive and Sweet Pepper Frittata, 28–29
    Loaded Smoked Salmon Breakfast Casserole, 75–76
    Moroccan Spiced Chicken with Sweet Potato Hash, 88–89
    Roasted Vegetable Mélange, 175
    Salmon Provençal, 144
    Sirloin with Sweet Bell Peppers, 83
    Skillet Cod with Fresh Tomato Salsa, 141
    Spicy Broccoli-Shrimp Farfalle, 138–139
    Spicy Split Pea Tabbouleh, 170
    Tabbouleh Pita Sandwich, 84
    Tuna Couscous Bowl with Grilled Vegetables, 61–62
Peppers, jalapeño
    California Egg White Scramble, 97
Peppers, roasted red
    Asparagus, Apple, and Feta Cheese Omelet, 51–52
    Chicken-Lentil Bowl with Roasted Red Pepper Dressing, 150–151
    Goat Cheese, Spinach, and Egg Frittata, 53
    Halibut with Olive-Tomato Sauce, 87
    Mediterranean Romaine Wedge Salad, 172
    Trout with Roasted Red Pepper Sauce, 63
Pesto
    Greek Vegetable and Herb Pinwheels, 77
    Green Vegetable Wrap with Basil Pesto, 31
    Pesto Vinaigrette, 190
    Whole-Wheat Spaghetti with Shrimp and Mint Pesto, 80–81
Pine nuts
    Balsamic-Basted Beef Kebabs with Barley and Spinach Risotto, 33–34
    Citrus-Artichoke Pesto with Vegetable Noodles, 58
    Couscous-Avocado Salad, 176–177
    Whole-Wheat Spaghetti with Shrimp and Mint Pesto, 80–81
Pistachios
    Moroccan Couscous Salad, 104–105
Plums
    Stone Fruit Overnight Bulgur, 72
Pomegranate juice
    Chia-Pomegranate Smoothie, 26
    Pomegranate Granita, 183
Pork
    Classic Pork Tenderloin Marsala, 157–158
    Rosemary-Citrus Roasted Pork Tenderloin, 159
Poultry, 7, 9
Proteins, 7, 9
Pumpkin purée
    Cranberry-Pumpkin Smoothie, 127
Pumpkin seeds
    Oatmeal Bowls with Blackberries, Seeds, and Honey, 124–125
    Quinoa Nuts and Seeds Overnight Porridge, 25

Q

Quinoa
    Chicken Shawarma Bowls, 112–113
    Oatmeal Bowls with Blackberries, Seeds, and
        Honey, 124–125
    Quinoa and Spinach Salad with Figs and Balsamic
        Dressing, 30
    Quinoa Nuts and Seeds Overnight Porridge, 25
    Quinoa-Walnut Pancakes, 128
    Shaved Cucumber Quinoa Bowl, 41
    Tabbouleh Pita Sandwich, 84

R

Radishes
    Salmon Bowl with Bulgur and Tahini Sauce,
        85–86
Relaxation, 11
Restaurants, 119
Rice
    Citrus-Chicken Vegetable "Risotto," 37–38
    Strawberry and Brown Rice Sunflower Seed
        Bowl, 126
    Wild Rice with Grapes, 167
Ricotta cheese
    Greek Vegetable and Herb Pinwheels, 77
Rosemary
    Rosemary-Citrus Roasted Pork Tenderloin, 159

S

Salads. See also Bowls
    Beet-Grapefruit Salad with Citrus-Basil Dressing,
        78–79
    Greek-Style Tuna Salad in Pita, 100
    Lemon-Spinach Salad with Pears and Blue Cheese,
        101–102
    Mashed Avocado Egg Salad with Crisps, 171
    Mediterranean Romaine Wedge Salad, 172
    Moroccan Couscous Salad, 104–105
    Quinoa and Spinach Salad with Figs and Balsamic
        Dressing, 30
    Roasted Brussels Sprouts and Halloumi Salad,
        173–174
    Salmon, Citrus, and Avocado Salad, 54
    Spicy Split Pea Tabbouleh, 170
Salmon
    Loaded Smoked Salmon Breakfast Casserole,
        75–76
    Salmon, Citrus, and Avocado Salad, 54
    Salmon Bowl with Bulgur and Tahini Sauce,
        85–86
    Salmon Provençal, 144

Salsas
    Fresh Tomato Salsa, 141
    Roasted Squash Salsa, 148–149
    White Bean Salsa, 142
Sandwiches and wraps
    Chickpea Veggie Burgers, 109
    Greek-Style Tuna Salad in Pita, 100
    Greek Vegetable and Herb Pinwheels, 77
    Green Vegetable Wrap with Basil Pesto, 31
    Grilled Vegetable Open-Faced Sandwich, 32
    Mashed Avocado Egg Salad with Crisps, 171
    Savory Hummus Breakfast Toasts, 50
    Sun-dried Tomato and Olive Tapenade with Goat
        Cheese Toasts, 55
    Tabbouleh Pita Sandwich, 84
Sardines
    Baked Sardine Patties, 143
Sauces. See also Dressings; Salsas
    Olive-Tomato Sauce, 87
    Roasted Red Pepper Sauce, 63
    Speedy Marinara Sauce, 191
    Tahini Sauce, 85–86
    Turkey-Tomato Ragù, 154
    Tzatziki Sauce, 192
    Yogurt-Mint Sauce, 65
Scallops
    Citrus-Herb Scallops, 137
Seeds, 7, 9, 16. See also specific
Shrimp
    Baking Sheet Spicy Shrimp with Vegetables, 108
    Simple Bouillabaisse, 39–40
    Spicy Broccoli-Shrimp Farfalle, 138–139
    Whole-Wheat Spaghetti with Shrimp and Mint
        Pesto, 80–81
Smoothies
    Avocado-Blueberry Smoothie, 96
    Chia-Pomegranate Smoothie, 26
    Cranberry-Pumpkin Smoothie, 127
    pre-prepping ingredients, 17
    Sweet Kale Smoothie, 49
Snacks
    Avocado on Multigrain Crackers, 23
    Balsamic Vinegar-Marinated Strawberries, 180
    Carrots and Hummus, 47
    Celery and Almond Butter, 23
    Cranberry-Pumpkin Seed Trail Mix, 93
    Feta Cheese with Watermelon Bites, 69
    Go Nuts, 69
    Hard-Boiled Eggs, 47
    Spiced Oranges with Dates, 185
    Tomato with Mozzarella Cheese, 93

Soups. *See also* Stews
    Beet-Fennel Soup with Goat Cheese, 82
    Tomato and Lentil Soup, 35
Spices, 7, 16–17
Spinach
    Asparagus, Apple, and Feta Cheese Omelet, 51–52
    Balsamic-Basted Beef Kebabs with Barley and
        Spinach Risotto, 33–34
    Barley Risotto with Sweet Potato and
        Spinach, 110
    Chicken Shawarma Bowls, 112–113
    Chickpea-Turkey Stew with Spinach, 155–156
    Goat Cheese, Spinach, and Egg Frittata, 53
    Greek Roasted Vegetable Bowl, 64
    Greek Vegetable and Herb Pinwheels, 77
    Green Vegetable Wrap with Basil Pesto, 31
    Lemon-Spinach Salad with Pears and Blue Cheese,
        101–102
    Quinoa and Spinach Salad with Figs and Balsamic
        Dressing, 30
    Roasted Brussels Sprouts and Halloumi Salad,
        173–174
    Tomato-Asparagus Omelets, 132–133
Split peas
    Spicy Split Pea Tabbouleh, 170
Squash. *See also* Zucchini
    Greek Roasted Vegetable Bowl, 64
    Pan-Fried Chicken with Roasted Squash Salsa,
        148–149
Stews
    Chickpea-Turkey Stew with Spinach, 155–156
    Simple Bouillabaisse, 39–40
Stress, 6
Sunflower seeds
    Overnight Steel-Cut Oats Porridge with
        Cherries, 95
    Quinoa and Spinach Salad with Figs and Balsamic
        Dressing, 30
    Strawberry and Brown Rice Sunflower Seed
        Bowl, 126
Sweet potatoes
    Barley Risotto with Sweet Potato and
        Spinach, 110
    Moroccan Spiced Chicken with Sweet Potato
        Hash, 88–89
    Roasted Vegetable Mélange, 175
Sweets
    Balsamic Vinegar-Marinated Strawberries, 180
    Creamy Panna Cotta, 184
    Fruit-Topped Meringues, 181
    Light Greek Yogurt Chocolate Pudding, 182

Pomegranate Granita, 183
    Spiced Oranges with Dates, 185
Swiss chard
    Egg-Stuffed Portobello Mushrooms, 129–130
    Egg White, Red Pepper, and Chard Scramble,
        73–74

T
Tahini
    Authentic Baba Ghanoush, 193–194
    Salmon Bowl with Bulgur and Tahini Sauce, 85–86
    Traditional Hummus, 188
30 minutes or less
    Avocado-Blueberry Smoothie, 96
    Baking Sheet Spicy Shrimp with Vegetables, 108
    Balsamic Vinegar-Marinated Strawberries, 180
    Black Olive and Sweet Pepper Frittata, 28–29
    Broiled Flounder with Nectarine and White Bean
        Salsa, 142
    Broiled Tomatoes with Feta, 165
    California Egg White Scramble, 97
    Chia-Pomegranate Smoothie, 26
    Chicken-Lentil Bowl with Roasted Red Pepper
        Dressing, 150–151
    Chili-Spiced Lamb Chops, 160
    Citrus-Herb Scallops, 137
    Classic Pork Tenderloin Marsala, 157–158
    Cranberry-Pumpkin Smoothie, 127
    Egg-Stuffed Portobello Mushrooms, 129–130
    Egg White, Red Pepper, and Chard Scramble,
        73–74
    Fresh Fruit Crumble Muesli, 71
    Goat Cheese, Spinach, and Egg Frittata, 53
    Golden Oatmeal Pancakes, 27
    Greek Breakfast Tostadas, 131
    Greek Herbed Beef Meatballs, 161
    Greek-Style Tuna Salad in Pita, 100
    Greek Vegetable and Herb Pinwheels, 77
    Green Vegetable Wrap with Basil Pesto, 31
    Halibut with Wilted Kale and Cherry Tomatoes, 36
    Hummus-Crusted Halibut, 103
    Kalamata Olive and Sweet Pepper Frittata, 28–29
    Lemon-Spinach Salad with Pears and Blue Cheese,
        101–102
    Mashed Avocado Egg Salad with Crisps, 171
    Mediterranean Romaine Wedge Salad, 172
    Oatmeal Bowls with Blackberries, Seeds, and
        Honey, 124–125
    Parmesan-Sautéed Zucchini with Spaghetti, 166
    Pesto Vinaigrette, 190
    Quinoa-Walnut Pancakes, 128

30 minutes or less *(continued)*
    Roasted Garlic, 189
    Salmon, Citrus, and Avocado Salad, 54
    Sautéed Dark Leafy Greens, 164
    Savory Hummus Breakfast Toasts, 50
    Sirloin with Sweet Bell Peppers, 83
    Skillet Cod with Fresh Tomato Salsa, 141
    Spiced Oranges with Dates, 185
    Sun-dried Tomato and Asparagus Frittata, 98–99
    Sun-dried Tomato and Olive Tapenade with Goat
        Cheese Toasts, 55
    Sweet Kale Smoothie, 49
    Tomato and Wine-Steamed Mussels, 136
    Tomato-Asparagus Omelets, 132–133
    Traditional Falafel, 168–169
    Traditional Hummus, 188
    Trout with Roasted Red Pepper Sauce, 63
    Trout with Ruby Red Grapefruit Relish, 145
    Tzatziki Sauce, 192
    Whole Baked Trout with Lemon and Herbs, 140
Tomatoes
    Broiled Tomatoes with Feta, 165
    California Egg White Scramble, 97
    Chicken-Lentil Bowl with Roasted Red Pepper
        Dressing, 150–151
    Chicken Shawarma Bowls, 112–113
    Chickpea-Turkey Stew with Spinach, 155–156
    Citrus-Chicken Vegetable "Risotto," 37–38
    Couscous-Avocado Salad, 176–177
    Halibut with Olive-Tomato Sauce, 87
    Halibut with Wilted Kale and Cherry Tomatoes, 36
    Mashed Avocado Egg Salad with Crisps, 171
    Mediterranean Romaine Wedge Salad, 172
    North African Chicken Apricot Tagine, 106–107
    Oven-Roasted Puttanesca with Ground Beef, 56–57
    Salmon Bowl with Bulgur and Tahini Sauce, 85–86
    Salmon Provençal, 144
    Shaved Cucumber Quinoa Bowl, 41
    Simple Bouillabaisse, 39–40
    Skillet Cod with Fresh Tomato Salsa, 141
    Speedy Marinara Sauce, 191
    Spicy Broccoli-Shrimp Farfalle, 138–139
    Spicy Split Pea Tabbouleh, 170
    Tabbouleh Pita Sandwich, 84
    Tomato and Lentil Soup, 35
    Tomato and Wine-Steamed Mussels, 136
    Tomato-Asparagus Omelets, 132–133
    Tomatoes Stuffed with Herbed Bulgur, 59–60
    Tuna Couscous Bowl with Grilled Vegetables,
        61–62
    Turkey-Tomato Ragù, 154

Tomatoes, sun-dried
    Greek Breakfast Tostadas, 131
    Greek Roasted Vegetable Bowl, 64
    Greek-Style Tuna Salad in Pita, 100
    Grilled Vegetable Open-Faced Sandwich, 32
    Oven-Roasted Puttanesca with Ground Beef, 56–57
    Savory Hummus Breakfast Toasts, 50
    Skillet Chicken Thighs with Bulgur and Feta,
        152–153
    Sun-dried Tomato and Asparagus Frittata, 98–99
    Sun-dried Tomato and Olive Tapenade with Goat
        Cheese Toasts, 55
Tools, 14–15
Trout
    Trout with Roasted Red Pepper Sauce, 63
    Trout with Ruby Red Grapefruit Relish, 145
    Whole Baked Trout with Lemon and Herbs, 140
Tuna
    Greek-Style Tuna Salad in Pita, 100
    Tuna Couscous Bowl with Grilled Vegetables, 61–62
Turkey
    Chickpea-Turkey Stew with Spinach, 155–156
    Turkey-Tomato Ragù, 154
Tzatziki sauce
    Chicken Shawarma Bowls, 112–113
    recipe, 192
    Tabbouleh Pita Sandwich, 84

V
Vegan
    Authentic Baba Ghanoush, 193–194
    Chia-Pomegranate Smoothie, 26
    Greek Roasted Vegetable Bowl, 64
    Moroccan Couscous Salad, 104–105
    Pesto Vinaigrette, 190
    Roasted Vegetable Mélange, 175
    Sautéed Dark Leafy Greens, 164
    Shaved Cucumber Quinoa Bowl, 41
    Speedy Marinara Sauce, 191
    Spiced Oranges with Dates, 185
    Spicy Split Pea Tabbouleh, 170
    Tomato and Lentil Soup, 35
    Tomatoes Stuffed with Herbed Bulgur, 59–60
    Traditional Falafel, 168–169
    Traditional Hummus, 188
    Wild Rice with Grapes, 167
Vegetables, 6, 9, 17. *See also specific*
    Grilled Vegetable Open-Faced Sandwich, 32
Vegetarian. *See also* Vegan
    Avocado-Blueberry Smoothie, 96
    Balsamic Vinegar-Marinated Strawberries, 180

Barley Risotto with Sweet Potato and Spinach, 110
Beet-Grapefruit Salad with Citrus-Basil Dressing, 78–79
Broiled Tomatoes with Feta, 165
California Egg White Scramble, 97
Chickpea Veggie Burgers, 109
Couscous-Avocado Salad, 176–177
Cranberry-Pumpkin Smoothie, 127
Egg-Stuffed Portobello Mushrooms, 129–130
Egg White, Red Pepper, and Chard Scramble, 73–74
Fresh Fruit Crumble Muesli, 71
Fruit-Topped Meringues, 181
Goat Cheese, Spinach, and Egg Frittata, 53
Golden Oatmeal Pancakes, 27
Greek Breakfast Tostadas, 131
Greek Vegetable and Herb Pinwheels, 77
Green Vegetable Wrap with Basil Pesto, 31
Grilled Vegetable Open-Faced Sandwich, 32
Kalamata Olive and Sweet Pepper Frittata, 28–29
Lemon-Spinach Salad with Pears and Blue Cheese, 101–102
Light Greek Yogurt Chocolate Pudding, 182
Mashed Avocado Egg Salad with Crisps, 171
Mediterranean Romaine Wedge Salad, 172
Oatmeal Bowls with Blackberries, Seeds, and Honey, 124–125
Overnight Steel-Cut Oats Porridge with Cherries, 95
Parmesan-Sautéed Zucchini with Spaghetti, 166
Pomegranate Granita, 183
Quinoa and Spinach Salad with Figs and Balsamic Dressing, 30
Quinoa Nuts and Seeds Overnight Porridge, 25
Quinoa-Walnut Pancakes, 128
Roasted Brussels Sprouts and Halloumi Salad, 173–174
Roasted Garlic, 189
Savory Hummus Breakfast Toasts, 50
Stone Fruit Overnight Bulgur, 72

Strawberry and Brown Rice Sunflower Seed Bowl, 126
Sun-dried Tomato and Asparagus Frittata, 98–99
Sweet Kale Smoothie, 49
Tabbouleh Pita Sandwich, 84
Tomato-Asparagus Omelets, 132–133
Tzatziki Sauce, 192

W
Walnuts
    Lemon-Spinach Salad with Pears and Blue Cheese, 101–102
    Quinoa-Walnut Pancakes, 128
Weight, 6, 11
Whole grains, 7, 9, 15. See also specific
Wine, 8
Wraps. See Sandwiches and wraps

Y
Yogurt, Greek
    Avocado-Blueberry Smoothie, 96
    Chicken with Yogurt-Mint Sauce, 65
    Fresh Fruit Crumble Muesli, 71
    Light Greek Yogurt Chocolate Pudding, 182
    Stone Fruit Overnight Bulgur, 72
    Sweet Kale Smoothie, 49
    Tzatziki Sauce, 192

Z
Zucchini
    Baking Sheet Spicy Shrimp with Vegetables, 108
    Citrus-Artichoke Pesto with Vegetable Noodles, 58
    Moroccan Spiced Chicken with Sweet Potato Hash, 88–89
    Parmesan-Sautéed Zucchini with Spaghetti, 166
    Roasted Vegetable Mélange, 175
    Tuna Couscous Bowl with Grilled Vegetables, 61–62
    Whole-Wheat Spaghetti with Shrimp and Mint Pesto, 80–81

ACKNOWLEDGMENTS

I would like to first and foremost thank God for being my strength and guide in writing this book. Without Him, I would not have had the wisdom or the physical ability to do so.

To my caring, loving, and supportive love, Brian: #MBHSFAEA.

My deep and sincere gratitude to my siblings and family for their continuous and unparalleled love, help, and support. Ada Fung, thank you for being my mentor during this journey—this would not be possible without you. A special thanks to Michelle Anderson and Therezia Alchoufete for your contribution and expertise and to the entire team at Callisto Media who helped make this book a success.

ABOUT THE AUTHOR

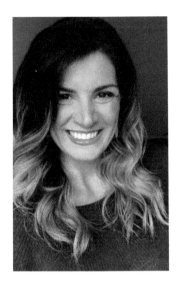

SUSAN ZOGHEIB was born in Beirut, Lebanon, and moved to the United States with her family in the late 1980s. She is a registered dietitian (RD) and holds a master's degree from Ryerson University in Toronto, Ontario, in nutrition communication. Susan is a food and nutrition expert and media consultant with more than 15 years of experience working as a clinical dietitian. In addition, she is a published author of four cookbooks, including a best-selling collection of renal diets and *The Mediterranean Diet Plan* cookbook. You can find her online at susueats.com, @susueats on Instagram, and facebook.com/susueats. She lives with her fiancé in Knoxville, Tennessee. In her spare time, she enjoys cooking, traveling, hiking, and running.

CPSIA information can be obtained
at www.ICGtesting.com
Printed in the USA
BVHW050319140919
558236BV00001B/1

9 781641 526302